WHAT TO EXPECT WHEN YOU ARE **EXPECTING** OR NOT EXPECTING... **AMPUTATION**

A Complete Guide to Amputation Recovery, Rehabilitation, Prosthetics, and Living Fully Again

—— **By Vaughan Debarr**

WHAT TO EXPECT WHEN YOU ARE EXPECTING OR NOT EXPECTING...AMPUTATION

Medical Disclaimer

The information in this book is for educational purposes only and does not constitute medical advice, diagnosis, or treatment. Always seek the advice of a qualified health provider regarding any medical condition or amputation recovery. Never disregard professional advice or delay in seeking it because of this book. Reliance on any information here is solely at your own risk.

Limit of Liability

The author makes no representations or warranties with respect to the accuracy or completeness of the contents and shall not be liable for any damages arising from the use of this book.

ISBN: [979-8-9958830-3-6]
Printed in the United States of America
First Edition: 2026

Dedication

This book is dedicated to every individual whose life has been touched by limb loss.

To the amputees—

Your strength is not defined by what was lost, but by how you continue to rise. Your courage, resilience, and determination inspire more people than you may ever realize.

To the practitioners and clinicians—

Thank you for your skill, your compassion, and your commitment to restoring mobility, independence, and dignity. The work you do changes lives every single day.

To the support staff and care teams—

Your behind-the-scenes dedication does not go unnoticed. You are an essential part of every patient's journey, offering stability, encouragement, and care when it matters most.

To the families and caregivers—

Your love, patience, and unwavering support are the foundation that helps others heal and move forward. You carry more than you show, and your presence makes all the difference.

And to everyone walking this path—

Whether you are just beginning or continuing your journey, know this:

You are not alone.

You are stronger than you think.

And your story is far from over.

With gratitude, respect, and hope—

this book is for you.

"Feet, what do I need you for when I have wings to fly?"

— Frida Kahlo

Your path may change,
but your strength, your courage, and your ability to move forward remain limitless.

Preface

This book was not written from theory.

It was written from experience.

There was a time when I didn't know what to expect—when the questions came faster than the answers, and the path forward felt uncertain. Each stage of my journey brought new challenges: physical, emotional, and mental. And with each step, I found myself wishing there was a guide—something honest, practical, and real—to help me understand what was ahead.

This is that guide.

My journey with limb loss did not happen all at once. It unfolded over time, beginning with a left below-knee amputation in 2013, progressing to a left above-knee amputation in 2017, and then becoming bilateral in 2019. Later that same year, I experienced a spinal stroke that resulted in paraplegia. Each moment brought its own set of obstacles—but also opportunities to learn, adapt, and grow.

Through it all, I came to understand something important:

Recovery is not just physical.

It is emotional.

It is mental.

And it is deeply personal.

Since entering the Orthotics and Prosthetics field in 2017, I've had the privilege of working alongside incredible clinicians, practitioners, and patients. I've seen firsthand the difference that education, preparation, and support can make. I've also seen the gaps—where people feel lost, overwhelmed, or unsure of what comes next.

This book was created to help fill those gaps.

Whether your amputation is planned or unexpected, whether you are a patient, a caregiver, or a professional, my goal is to provide you with clarity, guidance, and reassurance. You will find information here about what to expect physically, emotionally, and practically—but just as importantly, you will find encouragement.

This journey is not easy.

But it is possible.

You may not have chosen this path, but you can choose how you move forward.

Take this one step at a time.

Give yourself grace along the way.

And remember—you are not alone.

Forward

If you're holding this book, there's a good chance your life has changed—or is about to.

Maybe you've already had an amputation. Maybe you've just been told it's coming. Maybe you're here for someone you love. Wherever you are in this process, I want you to know something right away:

You are not alone.

I remember what those early days felt like—the questions, the fear, the uncertainty. The "What now?" and the "Why me?" that don't come with easy answers. It can feel like everything you knew about your life has shifted overnight.

That's why this book matters.

What makes this guide different is that it doesn't come from someone looking in from the outside. It comes from someone who has lived it—someone who understands not just the physical changes, but the emotional and mental weight that comes with them.

Vaughan's story is one of strength, but not in the way people often think. It's not about being fearless or having everything figured out. It's about continuing to move forward, even when things are uncertain. It's about learning, adapting, and finding your footing again—one step at a time.

As someone who has walked a similar path, I can tell you that information is important—but connection is what truly makes a difference. And this book offers both.

You'll find answers here.
You'll find guidance.
But more than anything, you'll find understanding.

There will be hard days. There will be moments that test you. But there will also be progress, growth, and victories—some small, some big—that remind you of what you're capable of.

This journey may not be one you chose.
But it is one you can learn to navigate.

And with the right support, the right mindset, and resources like this—you can move forward.

Keep going.
Take it one day at a time.

You're stronger than you think.

Foreword by:
Wendy Gamboa, Left Above Knee Amputee, Odessa, Texas

Forward II

There are books that inform, and there are books that transform. This is one of the rare works that does both.

What you are about to read is not simply a guide to amputation—it is a roadmap through one of life's most challenging and life-altering experiences. It speaks not only to the physical realities of limb loss, but also to the emotional, psychological, and deeply personal journey that follows.

What makes this book truly exceptional is its author.

Vaughan DeBarr brings something that cannot be taught in a classroom or learned from textbooks alone—lived experience. Her journey, marked by multiple amputations and a spinal stroke, is one of extraordinary resilience. Yet what stands out most is not just what she has endured, but how she has chosen to move forward—with strength, purpose, and a commitment to helping others do the same.

In my experience working with individuals facing limb loss, one of the greatest challenges is the uncertainty. Patients and families are often left asking, "What happens next?" This book answers that question with clarity, honesty, and compassion.

Vaughan bridges a critical gap between clinical knowledge and real-life experience. She understands the medical side of recovery through her work in the Orthotics & Prosthetics field, but more importantly, she understands what it feels like to live it—day by day, step by step.

This book will serve many audiences.

For patients, it offers reassurance, guidance, and a sense of direction during an overwhelming time.

For caregivers and families, it provides insight into how to support a loved one with empathy and understanding.

For practitioners, it is a reminder of the human side of the work we do—and the lasting impact of compassionate care.

Perhaps most importantly, this book offers something that is often difficult to find in the early stages of limb loss: hope.

Kevin Carroll, MS, CP, FAAOP (D)

An Expert in the O&P Field for over 40 years

Not unrealistic or superficial hope, but grounded, practical hope—the kind that comes from someone who has walked the path and continues to move forward with courage.

Vaughan's message is clear: life after limb loss is not the end of the story. It is a new chapter; one that can still be filled with purpose, growth, and possibility.

It is my honor to introduce this work and to recommend it to anyone navigating the journey of amputation, whether personally or professionally.

You are in capable hands.

TABLE OF CONTENTS

Dedication 4

Preface 7

Forward 9

Forward 2 11

Introduction 1

Chapter 1 Understanding Amputation 5

Chapter 2 "Why Me?" Navigating the First Wave of Questions .. 12

Chapter 3 Grief, Trauma, and the Psychology of Limb Loss 19

Chapter 4 Self-Care and Rebuilding Identity 26

Chapter 5 The Early Physical Recovery Phase 34

Chapter 6 Your Rehabilitation Team 42

Chapter 7 Choosing the Right Prosthetist 50

Chapter 8 Understanding Prosthetics 57

Chapter 9 Learning to Walk Again 65

Chapter 10 Strength, Balance, and Mobility 73

Chapter 11 Protecting Your Sound Limb 80

Chapter 12 You Are Not Alone 87

Chapter 13 Returning to Life 94

Chapter 14 Your New Normal 102

Chapter 15 The Long-Term Journey 109

Bonus Chapter For Caregivers and Loved Ones 116

Bonus Chapter Resources for New Lower Limb Amputees 123

Epilogue 131

Afterword 133

Acknowledgements 135

About the Author 137

Introduction

Welcome to Your New Journey

If you are reading this, your life has likely changed in a way you never expected.

Whether your amputation was sudden or something you had time to prepare for, the days and weeks surrounding it can feel overwhelming. You may be facing physical pain, emotional shock, uncertainty about the future, and questions that don't yet have clear answers. You may be wondering how life will look from here—or if it will ever feel "normal" again.

First, take a breath.

You are not alone. And while life may never look exactly the same as it once did, it can still be full, meaningful, independent, and even joyful.

This book was created to help guide you through that process.

Who This Book Is For

This book is written primarily for individuals who have experienced a lower limb amputation—whether recently or in the past—and are trying to understand what comes next.

It is also for:

- Those preparing for an upcoming amputation
- Family members, caregivers, and loved ones
- Anyone supporting someone through limb loss

Wherever you are in your journey—hospital bed, rehabilitation center, or back home trying to adjust—you will find information here that meets you where you are.

How to Use This Book

You do not need to read this book from beginning to end in order.

In fact, many people find it helpful to move between sections depending on what they're experiencing in the moment. Some days you may need emotional support and reassurance. Other days, you may be looking for practical guidance—how to care for your limb, what to expect in physical therapy, or how to choose a prosthetist.

Each chapter is designed to stand on its own while also building toward a bigger picture: helping you regain confidence, independence, and a sense of self.

Take your time. Revisit sections as needed. Skip ahead when it feels right.

This is your journey—there is no "correct" pace.

What This Book Will Help You Understand

Throughout these pages, you will learn about both the physical and emotional aspects of limb loss, including:

- What happens during and after an amputation
- How to navigate grief, trauma, and unexpected emotions
- How to care for your residual limb and prepare for a prosthesis
- What rehabilitation really looks like—and what progress feels like
- How to rebuild strength, balance, and mobility
- How to protect your remaining limb and long-term health
- How to reconnect with others and rebuild your life

Most importantly, you will begin to understand that recovery is not just about walking again—it is about learning how to live again.

A Word About What You May Be Feeling

There is no single "right way" to respond to limb loss.

You may feel:

- Shock or numbness
- Anger or frustration
- Fear about the future
- Grief for what was lost
- Determination to move forward
- Or all of these at once

Every one of these responses is valid.

Healing is not linear. Some days will feel like progress, and others may feel like setbacks. That does not mean you are failing—it means you are human, and you are adapting to something significant.

Words of Encouragement

It may be hard to believe right now, but people do adapt. People do rebuild. People do find strength they didn't know they had.

Over time, what feels impossible today can become manageable. What feels unfamiliar can become routine. And what feels like loss can gradually make space for growth.

You are still you.

Your identity, your worth, your potential—none of these were taken from you.

This journey will ask a lot of you. It will require patience, persistence, and self-compassion. But it will also reveal resilience, courage, and strength in ways you may never have experienced before.

You do not have to have everything figured out today.

You just have to take the next step—whatever that looks like for you.

And this book will be here to walk alongside you as you do.

Chapter 1

Understanding Amputation

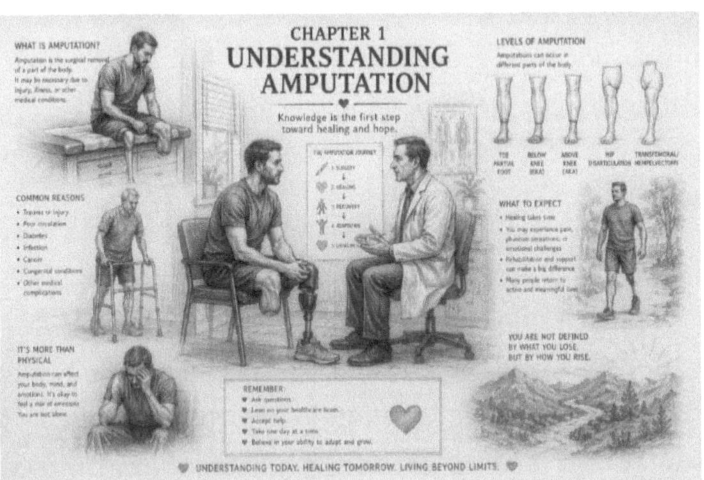

What Is an Amputation?

An amputation is the surgical removal of part or all of a limb. In this book, we are focusing on lower limb amputations, which involve the loss of a toe, foot, ankle, leg, or part of the hip.

Amputations are performed when a part of the body can no longer function properly or when keeping it would pose a serious risk to a person's overall health. While the idea of losing a limb can feel overwhelming, it is important to understand that amputation is often performed to save a life, relieve pain, or improve quality of life.

For many people, especially those who have been living with chronic pain, infection, or limited mobility, amputation can actually mark the beginning of relief and a new path forward.

Common Causes of Amputation

No two stories are exactly the same, but most lower limb amputations fall into several general categories:

Vascular Disease

This is the most common cause of lower limb amputation. Conditions such as poor circulation, peripheral artery disease, and complications from diabetes can reduce blood flow to the limbs. When tissues do not receive enough oxygen, they begin to break down, sometimes leading to non-healing wounds or infection.

Trauma

Severe injuries from car accidents, workplace incidents, or other accidents can result in damage that cannot be repaired. In these cases, amputation may be necessary either immediately or after attempts to save the limb are unsuccessful.

Infection

Serious infections—especially those that spread rapidly or affect the bone—can become life-threatening if not controlled. When infection cannot be contained, amputation may be the safest option.

Cancer

Certain types of cancer that affect the bone or soft tissue may require amputation to prevent the disease from spreading to other parts of the body.

Congenital Conditions

Some individuals are born with limb differences that may require surgical amputation to improve function or allow for prosthetic use.

Types of Lower Limb Amputations

Amputations are typically described based on where they occur on the limb. Understanding these terms can help you better communicate with your healthcare team.

Toe and Partial Foot Amputations

These involve the removal of one or more toes or parts of the foot. While they may seem minor compared to higher-level amputations, they can still significantly affect balance and walking.

Below-Knee Amputation (Transtibial)

This type involves removal of the lower leg below the knee. The knee joint remains intact, which is important because it allows for more natural movement and often easier rehabilitation with a prosthesis.

Above-Knee Amputation (Transfemoral)

In this case, the leg is removed above the knee joint. Because the knee is no longer present, walking with a prosthesis typically requires more energy and training.

Hip Disarticulation and Hemipelvectomy

These are less common and involve removal of the entire leg at the hip joint or part of the pelvis. Rehabilitation can be more complex, but independence is still possible with the right support and training.

What to Expect Surgically

If your amputation has already occurred, this section may help you better understand what your body has gone through. If your surgery is upcoming, it may help you feel more prepared.

Before Surgery

If the amputation is planned, your medical team may:

- Perform imaging and tests
- Discuss the level of amputation
- Talk with you about rehabilitation and prosthetic options
- Prepare you physically and emotionally for the procedure

In emergency situations, there may be little time for preparation. This can make the emotional impact more intense afterward, which is completely normal.

During Surgery

The surgeon removes the damaged tissue while preserving as much healthy bone and muscle as possible. Special care is taken to:

- Shape the residual limb for future prosthetic use
- Protect nerves to reduce pain complications
- Close the wound in a way that promotes healing

The goal is not just to remove what is damaged, but to create the best possible outcome for recovery and mobility.

After Surgery

After the procedure, you can expect:

- Hospital stay for monitoring and recovery
- Pain management (which may include medication and other techniques)
- Wound care and bandaging
- Early movement and positioning to prevent complications

You may also begin to experience something called phantom limb sensation, where it feels like the limb is still present. This is very common and will be discussed in more detail in a later chapter.

What Recovery Begins to Look Like

Recovery does not happen all at once—it unfolds in stages.

In the early days, the focus is on healing:

- Protecting the surgical site
- Managing pain

- Preventing infection
- Beginning gentle movement

As healing progresses, attention shifts toward:

- Strengthening your body
- Learning how to move safely
- Preparing for a prosthesis, if that is part of your plan

It is important to understand that recovery timelines vary widely. Factors such as overall health, level of amputation, and access to care all play a role.

There is no "normal" timeline—only your timeline.

Common Early Concerns

Many people share similar worries in the early stages:

- "Will I be able to walk again?"
- "How long will this take?"
- "What will my life look like now?"

These questions are valid—and they may not have immediate answers.

What matters most right now is not having everything figured out, but focusing on the next step in front of you. Over time, clarity comes through experience, support, and progress.

A Foundation for Moving Forward

Understanding what has happened to your body is one of the first steps in regaining a sense of control.

Amputation is not the end of your story—it is a turning point.

While there will be challenges ahead, there will also be solutions, support, and moments of progress that remind you of what is still possible.

In the next chapter, we will begin to explore one of the most common and difficult questions people face after limb loss: "Why me?"—and how to navigate the emotions that come with it.

Chapter 2

"Why Me?" Navigating the First Wave of Questions

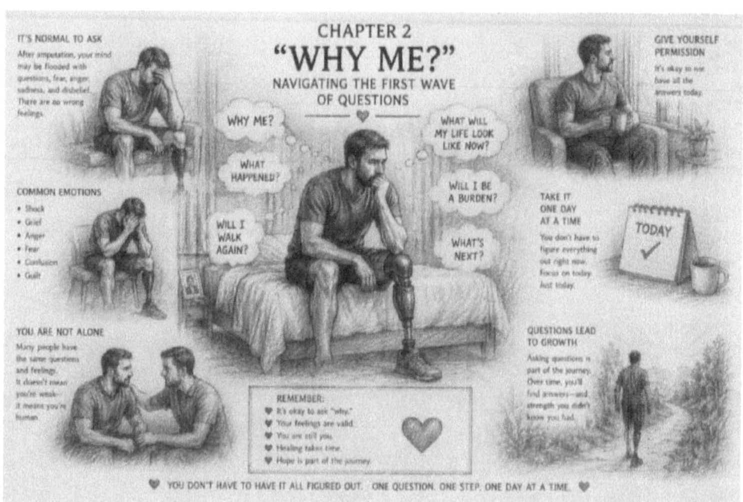

Processing Shock and Disbelief

When limb loss enters your life, one of the first reactions is often shock.

Even if your amputation was planned, discussed, and medically necessary, the moment it becomes real can feel disorienting. You may look down and expect to see what was once there. Your mind may struggle to reconcile what you know with what you feel.

This is not denial—it's your brain protecting you.

Shock acts as a buffer, giving you time to absorb a life-altering change in manageable pieces. You might feel numb, detached, or strangely calm. Or you may swing quickly between disbelief and intense emotion.

Common thoughts during this phase include:

- "This doesn't feel real."
- "I'll wake up and this will be over."
- "How is this my life now?"

There is no "correct" way to respond. Some people cry immediately. Others don't cry at all. Some want to talk; others withdraw.

All of it is valid.

Give yourself permission to process this at your own pace. You are not expected to have clarity right now. In fact, confusion is part of the process.

Guilt, Anger, and "What Ifs"

As the initial shock begins to settle, a wave of more complex emotions often follows.

Anger can show up in many directions:

- Anger at your body for "failing" you
- Anger at doctors, circumstances, or timing
- Anger at how unfair this feels

You may also experience guilt, especially if your amputation was related to a chronic condition, lifestyle factors, or an accident.

Thoughts might sound like:

- "If I had taken better care of myself..."

- "If I had made a different decision..."
- "This is my fault."

Then come the "what ifs."

What if you had caught it sooner?
What if you had chosen a different treatment?
What if things had gone differently that day?

These thoughts are powerful—and exhausting.

Here's the hard truth:
You cannot change the past, no matter how many times you replay it.

But here's the important truth:
These thoughts are a natural attempt to regain control.

Your mind is searching for logic in something that feels chaotic. It's trying to create a sense of order by asking, "Could this have been prevented?"

The problem is that staying stuck in this loop can keep you anchored in pain.

A helpful shift is not to suppress these thoughts—but to gently challenge them.

Instead of:
"I should have known better."

Try:
"I made the best decisions I could with what I knew at the time."

Instead of:
"This is my fault."

Try:
"This is my reality—and I can decide what comes next."

This isn't about dismissing responsibility. It's about releasing yourself from punishment.

Reframing the Narrative

At some point—slowly, and often unevenly—you may begin to notice a shift.

It might be subtle at first.

A moment where you think less about why this happened and more about what now?

Reframing your narrative is not about forced positivity. It is not about pretending everything is okay when it's not.

It's about reclaiming authorship of your story.

Right now, it may feel like something was taken from you—and that's true. But your story is not defined solely by loss.

You still have agency.

Reframing can begin with small mental adjustments:

- From "My life is over" → "My life is different"
- From "I can't do anything anymore" → "I will learn new ways to do things"
- From "I've lost everything" → "I still have things that matter—and I can build more"

These shifts are not instant. They are practiced.

And they don't erase grief—they exist alongside it.

You can feel sadness and determination.
You can feel anger and hope.

Both can be true at the same time.

The Power of Forward-Focused Thinking

One of the most important transitions in this stage is moving from past-focused thinking to forward-focused thinking.

This doesn't mean ignoring what happened. It means choosing not to live there permanently.

Forward-focused thinking sounds like:

- "What is one small thing I can do today?"
- "What does progress look like this week?"
- "Who can support me right now?"

Early on, progress may be incredibly small:

- Sitting up longer than yesterday
- Asking a question, you were afraid to ask
- Letting someone help you

These are not minor wins—they are foundational ones.

Momentum builds from small steps.

You Don't Have to Have the Answers Yet

There is pressure—both internal and external—to "figure things out."

People may ask:

- "What's your plan?"

- "When will you get a prosthetic?"
- "What's next?"

The honest answer, especially early on, is often:
"I don't know yet."

And that's okay.

You are allowed to be in a space of uncertainty. You are allowed to take time to understand your body, your emotions, and your new reality.

Clarity comes with time, experience, and support—not urgency.

Finding Stability in the Unstable

When everything feels uncertain, grounding yourself becomes essential.

This can look like:

- Creating small daily routines
- Focusing on immediate next steps rather than long-term outcomes
- Staying connected to people you trust

Even simple structure—waking up at the same time, eating regular meals, attending appointments—can create a sense of control when life feels unpredictable.

Stability doesn't come from having all the answers.
It comes from building consistency in the present moment.

A Closing Thought

If you are asking "Why me?"—you are not alone.

Almost everyone on this path has asked the same question.

But over time, many find that the question changes.

Not because the original question is answered—but because a more useful one takes its place:

“What can I do with the life I still have?”

You don’t need to answer that today.

For now, it is enough to acknowledge where you are, feel what you feel, and take the next step—however small it may be.

That is how this journey begins.

Chapter 3

Grief, Trauma, and the Psychology of Limb Loss

IT'S OKAY TO GRIEVE
Losing a limb is a profound loss. Grief is a natural response. There is no right or wrong way to grieve.
CHAPTER 3
GRIEF, TRAUMA, AND THE PSYCHOLOGY OF LIMB LOSS
Your emotions are valid.
Your healing matters.
Your life can still be meaningful.
YOU ARE NOT WEAK
Reaching out for support is a sign of strength, not weakness.
EMOTIONS MAY COME IN WAVES
• Anger
• Fear
• Numbness
• Guilt
• Anxiety
• Relief
• Hope
ACKNOWLEDGE
FEEL
UNDERSTAND
ACCEPT
HEAL
HEALING IS NOT LINEAR
Some days feel heavier than others. There will be good days and hard days. Both are part of the journey.
TRAUMA IS REAL
The experience of amputation can be traumatic. It may affect your body, mind, and spirit. It's not just in your head— it's in your whole self.
REMEMBER:
Your feelings are valid.
You are more than your amputation.
It's okay to not be okay.
Healing takes time.
You are still becoming
WHAT HELPS
• Talk about it
• Write it out
• Move your body
• Connect with others
• Practice self-compassion
• Allow joy to return
GRIEF IS THE PRICE WE PAY FOR LOVE. HEALING IS HOW WE HONOR LIFE.

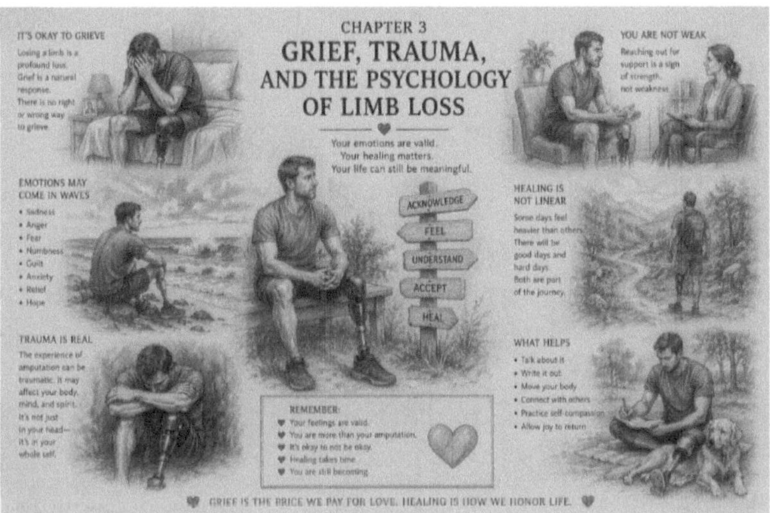

Grieving Your Limb

Grief after amputation is not only real—it is expected.

You have experienced a loss. Not just physical, but deeply personal. Your limb was part of how you moved through the world, how you completed everyday tasks, and how you understood your own body.

Grief may show up in ways you don't anticipate:

- Sadness that comes in waves
- Moments of longing for how things used to feel
- Emotional reactions to memories, routines, or even dreams

You may grieve:

- Your independence
- Your physical abilities
- Your identity as you once knew it

Some people feel this grief immediately. Others experience it weeks or months later, once the reality of daily life settles in.

There is no timeline. There is no "right way" to grieve.

You may have heard of the stages of grief—denial, anger, bargaining, depression, and acceptance—but in reality, grief is not linear. You might feel acceptance one day and deep sadness the next.

That doesn't mean you're going backward.

It means you're human.

Grief and the Body

Grief is not just emotional—it is physiological.

You may notice:

- Fatigue or low energy
- Changes in appetite
- Difficulty sleeping
- Trouble concentrating

Your nervous system is processing a major disruption. Healing requires energy, and your body is allocating resources to both physical recovery and emotional adaptation.

Be mindful of this: exhaustion doesn't always mean weakness—it often means your system is working hard behind the scenes.

PTSD and Medical Trauma

For many, amputation is not just a surgery—it is a traumatic event.

Whether your experience involved emergency care, prolonged hospitalization, or complications, your brain may interpret it as a threat that needs to be remembered and avoided.

This can lead to symptoms of post-traumatic stress:

- Intrusive memories or flashbacks
- Nightmares
- Hypervigilance (feeling constantly on edge)
- Avoidance of medical environments or reminders

You may find yourself reacting strongly to things that didn't bother you before—hospital smells, certain sounds, or even conversations about your experience.

This is your brain trying to protect you.

It has learned: This was dangerous. Stay alert.

The challenge is that this response can persist even when you are no longer in danger.

Recognizing this is important. These reactions are not irrational—they are adaptive responses that have simply outlasted their usefulness.

Depression, Anxiety, and Isolation

Emotional distress after limb loss is common—and often under-discussed.

Depression may feel like:

- A loss of motivation
- Persistent sadness or numbness
- Disconnection from things you once enjoyed

Anxiety may show up as:

- Fear about the future
- Worry about mobility, independence, or finances
- Overthinking or difficulty relaxing

Isolation can quietly develop alongside both.

You may feel:

- Different from others
- Misunderstood by people who haven't experienced limb loss
- Reluctant to be seen or social

Isolation can become a reinforcing cycle—the more disconnected you feel, the harder it becomes to reach out.

But connection is not optional in recovery—it is essential.

Even one supportive person—a friend, family member, therapist, or peer who understands—can make a measurable difference in emotional resilience.

Identity Disruption: "Who Am I Now?"

One of the most profound psychological impacts of limb loss is identity disruption.

Before this, you may not have consciously thought about your body as part of your identity—but now, it may feel central.

You might wonder:

- "Am I still the same person?"
- "How do others see me now?"
- "What does this mean for my future?"

These questions are not superficial—they are foundational.

Your identity is being restructured.

It's important to understand that identity is not fixed—it evolves. While something has changed, your corc values, personality, and capabilities still exist.

This phase is less about "getting back to who you were" and more about integrating who you are becoming.

When to Seek Help—and How

There is a misconception that you should "handle this on your own" or wait until things get severe before asking for help.

That approach is inefficient—and often harmful.

Consider seeking support if you notice:

- Persistent feelings of hopelessness
- Ongoing anxiety that interferes with daily function
- Withdrawal from people and activities

- Difficulty adjusting to your new reality

Support options include:

Mental Health Professionals

Psychologists, counselors, or therapists trained in trauma or medical adjustment can help you process what you've experienced and develop coping strategies.

Peer Support

Connecting with someone who has gone through limb loss can normalize your experience in a way few others can. They've been where you are.

Support Groups

Group environments—whether in-person or virtual—offer shared understanding, practical advice, and emotional validation.

Seeking help is not a sign that you're struggling more than you should.

It's a sign that you are taking your recovery seriously.

Building Emotional Resilience

Resilience is often misunderstood as toughness or the absence of struggle.

In reality, resilience is your ability to adapt, recover, and continue moving forward—even while experiencing difficulty.

You build resilience by:

- Allowing yourself to feel, rather than suppressing emotions
- Developing routines that support stability

- Staying connected to others
- Setting small, achievable goals

Resilience is not something you either have or don't have.

It is something you build—intentionally, over time.

A Closing Perspective

You have been through something significant.

The emotional weight of this experience deserves acknowledgment—not minimization.

Grief, trauma, anxiety, identity shifts—these are not side effects. They are central parts of the journey.

But they are not permanent states.

With time, support, and effort, the intensity of these feelings can change. They may not disappear entirely, but they can become more manageable, more integrated, and less overwhelming.

You are not expected to "be okay" right now.

You are only asked to keep going.

And that—especially in this phase—is more than enough.

Chapter 4

Self-Care and Rebuilding Identity

CHAPTER 4
SELF-CARE AND REBUILDING IDENTITY
You are more than what you've lost.
You are becoming who you're meant to be.
PUT YOURSELF FIRST
Self-care isn't selfish—it's essential. You can't pour from an empty cup.
CARE FOR YOUR BODY
Move your body in ways that feel good. Eat well. Rest deeply. Your body is your foundation.
NOURISH YOUR MIND
Your thoughts shape your reality. Practice gratitude. Challenge negativity. Choose hope.
REBUILD YOUR IDENTITY
You are not defined by your amputation.
Create a life that excites you.
SET BOUNDARIES
Protect your energy. It's okay to say no.
CELEBRATE PROGRESS
Every step forward matters. Honor your strength. You are making a difference in your own life.
ACCEPTANCE
GROWTH
PURPOSE
CONFIDENCE
HOPE
REMEMBER:
You are still you.
Your story isn't over.
Small steps create big change.
Be patient and kind with yourself.
You are worthy of a beautiful life.
YOU ARE NOT GOING BACK TO WHO YOU WERE.
YOU ARE MOVING FORWARD TO WHO YOU ARE MEANT TO BE.

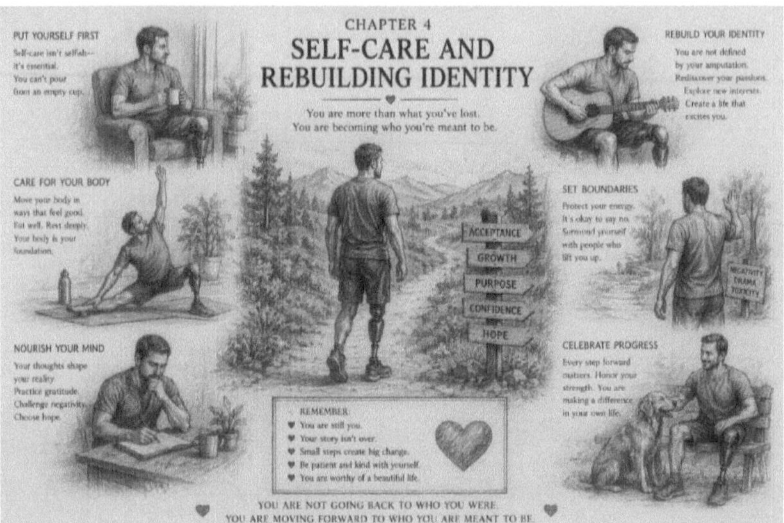

Self-Compassion in Practice

After limb loss, many people become harder on themselves—not kinder.

You may expect yourself to "bounce back," stay positive, or progress quickly. When that doesn't happen, frustration and self-criticism can take over.

But recovery—both physical and psychological—is not driven by pressure. It's supported by consistency, patience, and self-compassion.

Self-compassion is not indulgence. It is a disciplined way of treating yourself with the same respect you would offer someone else in your position.

In practice, it looks like:

- Acknowledging when something is difficult instead of minimizing it
- Allowing rest without labeling it as failure
- Replacing harsh internal dialogue with more accurate, supportive language

Instead of:
"I should be further along."

Try:
"I am progressing at a pace my body and mind can sustain."

Instead of:
"I'm weak for struggling with this."

Try:
"This is a major adjustment. Struggling is part of adapting."

Self-compassion creates psychological stability. Without it, recovery becomes unnecessarily adversarial—you against yourself.

Body Image and Confidence

Your relationship with your body may feel different now.

You may notice:

- Discomfort looking at your residual limb
- Reluctance to wear certain clothing

- Concern about how others perceive you

These reactions are common. Your body has changed, and your mind is adjusting to that change.

Confidence does not return by ignoring these feelings—it develops through gradual exposure and acceptance.

This might begin with small steps:

- Looking at your limb without avoidance
- Becoming familiar with touch and sensation
- Choosing clothing that makes you feel comfortable, not hidden

Over time, many people move from seeing their body as "damaged" to seeing it as "adapted."

Your body has been through something significant. It is not less—it is different.

And different does not eliminate value, capability, or strength.

Creating Healthy Routines

In the early phases of recovery, life can feel unpredictable. Medical appointments, physical limitations, and emotional fluctuations can disrupt your sense of structure.

Routines help restore control.

They do not need to be complex. In fact, simple, repeatable habits are more effective.

Start with foundational elements:

- Consistent sleep and wake times

- Regular meals
- Scheduled movement or therapy exercises
- Personal care routines

As your capacity increases, you can expand:

- Time outdoors
- Social interaction
- Structured rehabilitation goals

Routines serve two key functions:

1. They reduce decision fatigue during an already demanding period
2. They reinforce a sense of forward movement, even on difficult days

You may not control everything—but you can control your daily rhythm.

Reconnecting With Your Body

After amputation, it's common to feel disconnected from your body.

This can happen due to:

- Pain or discomfort
- Medical procedures
- Changes in sensation

Reconnection is a gradual process.

It may involve:

- Learning how your residual limb responds to touch and pressure
- Understanding new physical limits and capabilities
- Participating in physical therapy with intention, not just obligation

Movement becomes an important part of this process.

Even small actions—stretching, positioning, balance work—help rebuild trust between you and your body.

Instead of viewing your body as something that has failed you, you begin to experience it as something you can work with again.

Who Am I Now?

This question often emerges quietly, but persistently.

Before your amputation, parts of your identity may have been tied to:

- Physical ability
- Work or hobbies
- Independence

Now, those reference points may feel uncertain.

It's important to understand. identity is not erased, it is restructured.

You are still:

- The same person with the same values
- Capable of connection, growth, and contribution
- Able to build a meaningful life

But you may also become:

- More adaptable
- More aware of your resilience
- More intentional about how you live

This phase is not about returning to a previous version of yourself.

It is about integrating your experience into a new, expanded identity.

Letting Go of Comparison

One of the fastest ways to undermine your progress is comparison.

You may compare yourself to:

- Who you were before
- Other amputees who seem further along
- Expectations—your own or others'—about recovery timelines

Comparison creates unnecessary pressure and distorts reality.

Your recovery is influenced by:

- Your specific medical condition
- Your level of amputation
- Your support system
- Your mental and physical health

No two paths are identical.

Progress should be measured against your own starting point—not someone else's outcome.

Rebuilding Confidence Through Action

Confidence is often thought of as something you "feel" first.

In reality, it is usually built through action.

You regain confidence by:

- Attempting tasks—even when uncertain
- Practicing new skills repeatedly
- Experiencing small successes

Confidence is not required to begin.
It is the result of beginning.

This may look like:

- Standing longer than you did yesterday
- Completing part of a task independently
- Trying something new, even if it feels uncomfortable

Each action reinforces capability. Over time, capability builds confidence.

A Closing Perspective

Rebuilding yourself after limb loss is not a single step—it is an ongoing process.

There will be moments of doubt, frustration, and fatigue. That does not mean you are failing.

It means you are actively adapting.

Self-care is not separate from recovery—it is a core component of it.
Your identity is not lost—it is evolving.

You do not need to have a complete picture of who you are becoming.

You only need to continue showing up, taking care of yourself, and allowing that identity to take shape—one day at a time.

Chapter 5

The Early Physical Recovery Phase

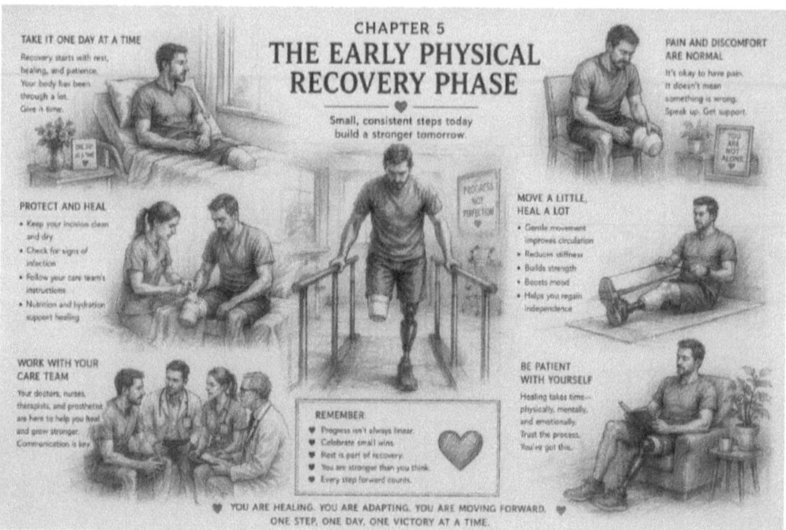

The early phase of recovery is where healing begins—both visibly and beneath the surface.

This stage can feel slow, uncomfortable, and at times frustrating. Progress may not always be obvious, and setbacks can happen. But this phase is critical. The way your residual limb heals and adapts now will directly impact your comfort, mobility, and long-term prosthetic success.

Think of this as your foundation. What you do here matters.

Wound Healing and Residual Limb Care

After surgery, your primary focus is healing.

Your residual limb (often called a "residuum") needs time to recover from both the procedure and the trauma your body has experienced.

Key priorities during this phase include:

- Keeping the incision clean and dry
- Monitoring for signs of infection (redness, warmth, drainage, unusual odor, fever)
- Following all medical instructions closely

Healing timelines vary depending on your health, circulation, and the reason for amputation. Some people heal relatively quickly; others require more time and monitoring.

You may also notice:

- Swelling (edema)
- Sensitivity or tenderness
- Changes in skin texture

All of these are normal to a degree.

Your care team will guide you on:

- When bandages can be removed
- When gentle handling is appropriate
- When you can begin preparing for prosthetic use

This is not the stage to rush. Proper healing now prevents complications later.

Shrinkers, Shaping, and Desensitization

As your incision heals, attention shifts to shaping your residual limb.

This process is essential for future prosthetic fit.

Shrinkers or compression garments are often introduced to:

- Reduce swelling
- Help shape the limb into a more functional form
- Improve circulation

Consistent use is important. Irregular use can slow progress and affect how well a prosthetic socket will fit later.

Desensitization is another key component.

After amputation, your limb may be extremely sensitive—or in some areas, feel numb.

Desensitization techniques help your nervous system adapt. These may include:

- Light tapping or massage
- Rubbing different textures over the skin
- Gentle pressure application

At first, even light touch may feel uncomfortable. Over time, with consistent exposure, your tolerance improves.

The goal is to make your limb more comfortable for contact—especially important when wearing a prosthesis.

Phantom Limb Sensation & Pain

One of the most unexpected experiences after amputation is phantom limb sensation.

You may feel as though your limb is still there.

This can include:

- Tingling
- Pressure
- Movement sensations

This is normal.

Your brain still has a "map" of your limb, and it takes time to adjust.

Phantom limb pain, however, is different.

It can feel like:

- Sharp or shooting pain
- Burning or cramping
- Twisting or unnatural positioning

Not everyone experiences phantom pain, but many do at some point.

Management strategies may include:

- Medications prescribed by your doctor
- Mirror therapy
- Desensitization techniques
- Physical therapy interventions

It's important to communicate openly about your symptoms. Phantom pain is real—and treatable.

Positioning and Contracture Prevention

During early recovery, how you position your body matters more than you might expect.

If certain muscles remain shortened for too long, you can develop contractures—permanent tightening that limits movement.

For example:

- Keeping a knee constantly bent can make it difficult to fully straighten later
- Staying in one position too often can restrict mobility

Your care team or therapist will guide you on:

- Proper positioning
- Stretching routines
- Safe ways to sit, lie, and move

Prevention is significantly easier than correction.

Volume Changes and What They Mean

Your residual limb will not stay the same size.

In fact, volume changes are expected—especially in the early months.

You may notice:

- Rapid decreases in swelling
- Daily fluctuations depending on activity level

- Changes in how your limb feels inside compression garments

These changes are a normal part of healing.

However, they also impact prosthetic fitting. A limb that is still changing significantly may not yet be ready for a permanent prosthesis.

This is why early fittings are often temporary or adjustable.

Understanding this can help manage expectations:

- Fit will not be perfect right away
- Adjustments will be frequent
- Patience is required

This is not a setback—it is part of the process.

Pain vs. Healing: Knowing the Difference

Not all discomfort is the same.

Learning to distinguish between expected healing sensations and potential problems is important.

Common, expected sensations:

- Mild to moderate soreness
- Sensitivity to touch
- Occasional sharp or tingling feelings

Warning signs to report:

- Increasing pain rather than gradual improvement
- Significant swelling or redness
- Signs of infection

- Skin breakdown

When in doubt, communicate with your care team.

Early intervention prevents complications.

Building Early Mobility

Even before prosthetic use, movement matters.

Depending on your situation, this may include:

- Sitting balance exercises
- Transfers (bed to chair, chair to wheelchair)
- Upper body strengthening
- Use of assistive devices

Early mobility helps:

- Maintain strength
- Improve circulation
- Support mental well-being

Progress may feel slow—but every movement contributes to your recovery.

A Closing Perspective

This phase is not the most visible or exciting part of recovery—but it is one of the most important.

Healing. Shaping. Adapting.

These are the building blocks for everything that follows.

You may not feel like you're making big strides yet—but you are laying the groundwork for future independence and mobility.

Stay consistent. Stay patient. Stay engaged with your care.

Your progress is happening—even when it's not immediately obvious.

Chapter 6

Your Rehabilitation Team

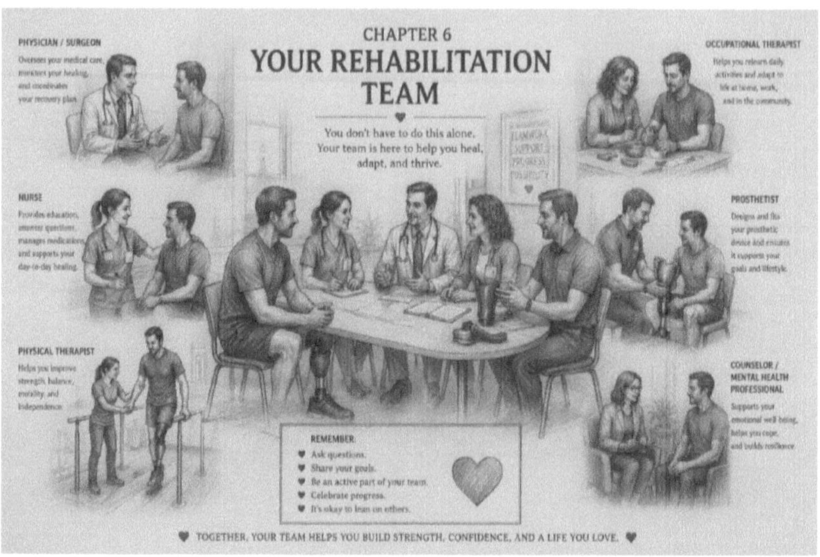

Recovery after limb loss is not a solo effort. It is a coordinated process involving multiple professionals, each with a specific role in helping you regain function, independence, and confidence.

Understanding who is on your team—and how to work with them—can significantly improve your outcomes.

You are not just a patient in this process. You are an active participant.

Who Makes Up Your Rehabilitation Team?

Your rehabilitation team may include several specialists, depending on your needs and stage of recovery. While titles and roles can vary slightly, the core team typically includes:

- Prosthetist
- Physical Therapist (PT)
- Occupational Therapist (OT)
- Physician or surgeon
- Mental health professional
- Case manager or care coordinator
- Peer mentor

Each plays a distinct role, but the most effective recovery happens when these roles work together—and when you are engaged in the process.

The Prosthetist: Your Prosthetic Specialist

Your prosthetist is responsible for designing, fitting, and adjusting your prosthesis.

Their role includes:

- Evaluating your residual limb
- Recommending appropriate prosthetic components
- Creating and modifying your socket (the part that connects your limb to the prosthesis)
- Making ongoing adjustments as your limb changes

A strong prosthetist-patient relationship is critical. Fit, comfort, and function are not one-time decisions—they evolve over time.

You should feel comfortable:

- Asking questions
- Reporting discomfort
- Requesting adjustments

A well-fitting prosthesis is not a luxury—it is essential for mobility and long-term health.

Physical Therapy (PT): Movement and Mobility

Your physical therapist focuses on helping you regain strength, balance, and mobility.

PT typically includes:

- Strength training
- Balance and coordination exercises
- Gait training (learning to walk with or without a prosthesis)
- Fall prevention strategies

Physical therapy is where much of the functional progress happens.

It can also be challenging.

You may feel:

- Fatigued
- Frustrated with slow progress
- Discouraged by setbacks

This is normal.

Consistency is more important than intensity. Showing up, even on difficult days, is what drives progress.

Occupational Therapy (OT): Daily Living and Independence

While PT focuses on movement, occupational therapy focuses on function—how you perform everyday activities.

OT may help you:

- Dress, bathe, and groom independently
- Modify your home or workspace
- Learn adaptive techniques for daily tasks
- Use assistive devices effectively

The goal is practical independence.

Small improvements in daily tasks often have a large impact on confidence and quality of life.

Mental Health Support: The Psychological Component

Recovery is not just physical.

A mental health professional—such as a psychologist, counselor, or therapist—can help you:

- Process grief and trauma
- Manage anxiety or depression
- Develop coping strategies
- Navigate identity changes

This support is often underutilized—but it is one of the most important components of long-term success.

You do not need to wait until you are struggling significantly to seek support. Early engagement can make the entire process more manageable.

Case Managers and Care Coordinators

Healthcare systems can be complex.

A case manager or care coordinator helps ensure that:

- Your services are organized
- Appointments are scheduled efficiently
- Insurance processes are handled appropriately
- Communication between providers is maintained

They act as a logistical bridge, allowing you to focus more on recovery and less on administrative challenges.

If you have access to one, use them.

Peer Mentors: Lived Experience Matters

One of the most valuable resources in your recovery may be someone who has already walked this path.

A peer mentor is typically:

- Another amputee
- Someone further along in their recovery
- Someone trained to provide guidance and support

They offer something no textbook or clinical training can fully provide, real experience.

They can help you:

- Set realistic expectations
- Navigate challenges
- See what is possible

Perhaps most importantly, they provide proof that progress—and a full life—is achievable.

How the Team Works Together

Ideally, your rehabilitation team communicates and collaborates.

For example:

- Your physical therapist may provide feedback to your prosthetist about gait issues
- Your prosthetist may adjust your device based on therapy performance
- Your physician monitors your overall health and healing

When communication is strong, your care becomes more efficient and effective.

However, coordination is not always automatic.

This is where your role becomes important.

Advocating for Yourself

You are the only constant in your care.

Providers may change. Schedules may shift. Systems may not always be seamless.

Advocating for yourself means:

- Asking questions when something is unclear
- Speaking up if something doesn't feel right
- Requesting adjustments when needed
- Ensuring your concerns are addressed

You do not need medical expertise to advocate effectively. You only need to be engaged and willing to communicate.

Examples of self-advocacy:

- "This prosthesis feels uncomfortable after an hour—can we adjust it?"
- "I'm struggling with this exercise—can we modify it?"
- "I don't feel like my concerns are being addressed—what are my options?"

Your feedback is not an inconvenience—it is essential data.

Building Trust with Your Team

Strong outcomes depend on trust.

Trust is built through:

- Clear communication
- Consistency
- Mutual respect

Be honest about your experiences—even when they're frustrating or discouraging.

Your team is there to help, but they can only respond to what they know.

At the same time, evaluate your team.

You should feel:

- Heard
- Respected
- Supported

If you consistently feel dismissed or overlooked, it may be appropriate to explore other providers.

A Closing Perspective

Recovery is not something you navigate alone—even though it may feel that way at times.

Your rehabilitation team exists to support, guide, and equip you. Each member contributes a piece of the overall process.

But the most important member of that team is you.

Your effort, your communication, and your willingness to engage will shape your outcomes more than any single intervention.

You don't need to know everything.
You don't need to do everything perfectly.

You just need to stay involved, stay informed, and continue moving forward—one step, one session, one interaction at a time.

Chapter 7

Choosing the Right Prosthetist

CHAPTER 7
CHOOSING THE RIGHT PROSTHETIST
The right prosthetist makes all the difference in your comfort, confidence, and independence.
EXPERIENCE MATTERS
Look for a prosthetist who is certified, experienced, and specializes in your level of amputation and activity goals.
COMMUNICATION IS KEY
They should listen to your goals, answer your questions, and explain things clearly.
CUSTOMIZED CARE
Your prosthesis should be customized to your body, lifestyle and long-term goals—not one size-fits-all.
TECHNOLOGY AND OPTIONS
A good prosthetist offers the latest technology and explains your options without pressure.
ONGOING SUPPORT
Your needs will change. Choose someone who provides follow-up care and adjusts your prosthesis as you grow stronger.
TRUST YOUR INSTINCTS
You should feel comfortable, respected, and confident in your prosthetist and their team.
QUESTIONS TO ASK
Are you certified and licensed?
How many amputees do you work with?
What experience do you have with my level of amputation?
What options are best for my lifestyle and goals?
How do you handle follow-up care and adjustments?
Will my insurance cover your services?
THE RIGHT PROSTHETIST IS MORE THAN A PROVIDER—THEY ARE YOUR PARTNER IN RECOVERY AND IN LIFE.

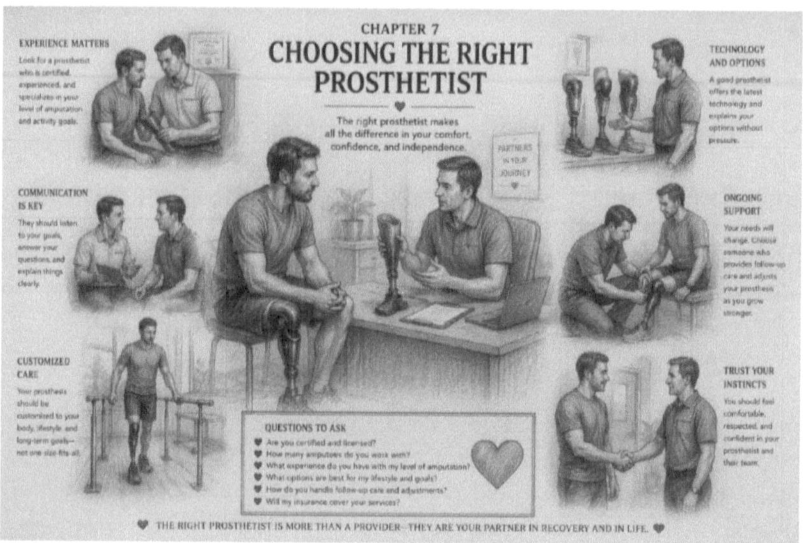

Selecting a prosthetist is one of the most important decisions you will make in your recovery.

This is not a one-time interaction. Your prosthetist will be a long-term partner in your mobility, comfort, and independence. The quality of that relationship—and their technical skill—will directly affect how well your prosthesis fits, how it functions, and how you feel using it.

Not all prosthetists are the same.

And you have the right to choose.

What Matters Most

When evaluating a prosthetist, technical ability is essential—but it is not the only factor.

You are looking for a combination of:

- Clinical expertise
- Communication skills
- Responsiveness
- Willingness to individualize your care

A strong prosthetist will:

- Take time to understand your lifestyle and goals
- Explain options clearly, without rushing
- Make adjustments proactively, not reactively
- Treat you as a partner—not just a case

Your prosthesis is not just a device. It is something you will rely on daily. Precision and personalization matter.

Experience and Specialization

Not every prosthetist has the same level of experience with every type of amputation.

It is reasonable—and important—to ask:

- How many patients like me have you worked with?
- Do you specialize in upper or lower limb prosthetics?
- What experience do you have with my level of amputation?

Experience does not guarantee perfection, but it often leads to more efficient problem-solving and better outcomes.

If your goals include high activity levels, work-specific demands, or adaptive sports, your prosthetist should have experience supporting those outcomes.

Questions to Ask

You are not expected to know everything—but asking the right questions helps you evaluate fit and competence.

Consider asking:

About Approach

- "How do you determine the right prosthetic setup for someone like me?"
- "What is your process for fitting and adjustments?"

About Expectations

- "What should I expect in the first 3–6 months?"
- "How often will adjustments be needed?"

About Support

- "If I have a problem, how quickly can I be seen?"
- "Do you coordinate with my physical therapist?"

About Outcomes

- "What challenges do patients like me typically face?"
- "How do you handle fit issues or discomfort?"

The goal is not to test them—it is to understand how they think, communicate, and problem-solve.

Communication Style Matters

Technical skill is critical. But communication is what makes that skill usable.

You should feel comfortable:

- Asking questions without hesitation
- Describing discomfort honestly
- Requesting changes

A prosthetist who listens carefully and explains clearly will be far more effective than one who is technically skilled but difficult to communicate with.

If you leave appointments feeling confused, rushed, or dismissed, that is a concern.

You need clarity—not uncertainty.

Warning Signs

Not every provider will be the right fit. Pay attention to red flags.

These may include:

- Rushing through appointments
- Dismissing your concerns or discomfort
- Offering limited options without explanation
- Reluctance to make adjustments
- Poor follow-up or difficulty scheduling

Another key warning sign: being told that discomfort is something you should simply "get used to."

A prosthesis may require adaptation—but persistent pain or poor fit should not be normalized.

Access and Availability

Even an excellent prosthetist is less effective if access is limited.

Consider:

- Location and travel distance
- Appointment availability
- Responsiveness to urgent issues

Early in your prosthetic journey, adjustments may be frequent. If it is difficult to be seen when needed, small issues can become larger problems.

Consistency of care matters.

Insurance and Patient Rights

Prosthetic care often involves insurance approvals, documentation, and cost considerations.

You should understand:

- What your insurance covers
- What documentation is required
- What your out-of-pocket responsibilities may be

A good prosthetic clinic will help guide you through this process—but you should remain informed.

You also have rights:

- The right to choose your provider

- The right to seek a second opinion
- The right to ask questions about cost and coverage

Do not assume you are locked into a single option.

Trial, Adjustment, and Iteration

Your first prosthesis will not be perfect.

Fit evolves as:

- Your residual limb changes
- Your activity level increases
- Your goals become clearer

A strong prosthetist expects this.

They approach prosthetic fitting as an ongoing process:

- Evaluate
- Fit
- Test
- Adjust
- Repeat

Your role is to provide accurate feedback. Their role is to translate that feedback into technical adjustments.

This is a collaborative system—not a one-time transaction.

Trusting Your Instincts

Beyond qualifications and logistics, there is a simpler question:

Do you trust this person?

Trust is built when:

- You feel heard
- Your concerns are taken seriously
- You are included in decisions

If something feels off, it is worth paying attention to.

You are not being difficult by asking for better care. You are being responsible for your long-term outcomes.

A Closing Perspective

Your prosthetist is not just providing a device—they are helping shape how you move through the world.

Take the time to choose carefully.

Ask questions. Evaluate options. Pay attention to how you are treated.

The right prosthetist will not only improve your physical comfort and mobility—they will also give you confidence in the process.

And confidence, especially in this stage of recovery, is a powerful advantage.

Chapter 8

Understanding Prosthetics

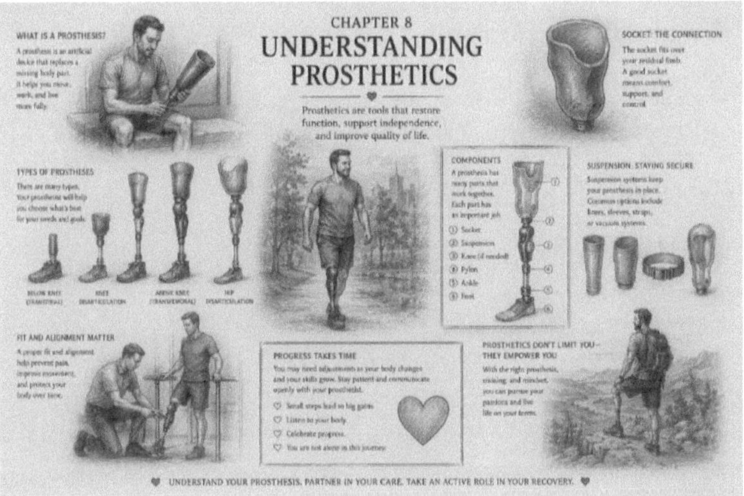

A prosthesis is more than a piece of equipment—it is a tool that allows you to regain function, independence, and mobility.

At first, prosthetics can feel complex and overwhelming. There are unfamiliar terms, multiple components, and a wide range of options. But understanding the basics will help you make informed decisions and communicate more effectively with your prosthetist.

You don't need to become an expert.
You do need to understand how your device works for you.

How a Prosthesis Works

At its core, a prosthesis is designed to replace the function of a missing limb.

For lower-limb amputees, that typically means:

- Supporting your body weight
- Providing stability
- Allowing efficient, controlled movement

For upper-limb amputees, it may involve:

- Grasping and releasing objects
- Assisting with daily tasks
- Restoring symmetry and function

A prosthesis works by transferring forces from your body through the device to the ground (or to an object, in the case of upper limbs). The goal is to create a system that feels as natural, stable, and efficient as possible.

But it's important to understand:

A prosthesis does not "replace" your limb in a biological sense. It is a mechanical system that you learn to use.

Mastery comes with time, practice, and proper fit.

Core Components of a Prosthesis

While designs vary, most prosthetic systems include several key components:

1. The Socket

This is the most important part of your prosthesis.

It is the custom-made interface between your residual limb and the device. A well-fitting socket:

- Distributes pressure evenly
- Minimizes pain and skin breakdown
- Provides control and stability

If the socket is not right, nothing else will feel right.

2. Suspension System

This is how the prosthesis stays attached to your body.

Common systems include:

- Suction or vacuum systems
- Pin-lock systems
- Straps or harnesses

Each has advantages and trade-offs related to comfort, security, and ease of use.

3. Structural Components (Pylons/Frames)

These connect the socket to the terminal device (foot, hand, etc.).

They provide:

- Support
- Alignment
- Adjustability

4. Terminal Device

This is the functional end of the prosthesis.

For lower limb:

- Prosthetic foot or knee systems

For upper limb:

- Hooks, hands, or myoelectric devices

This component plays a major role in how you move and interact with your environment.

Types of Prosthetic Options

Prosthetics are not one-size-fits-all. Your options will depend on your:

- Level of amputation
- Activity level
- Goals
- Medical condition

For lower limb prosthetics, options may include:

- Basic, stable feet for everyday walking
- Energy-storing feet for more dynamic movement
- Microprocessor-controlled knees for advanced mobility

For upper limb prosthetics, options may include:

- Body-powered systems (controlled by cables and movement)
- Myoelectric systems (controlled by muscle signals)
- Passive prosthetics (primarily cosmetic but functional for support)

Each option comes with trade-offs in cost, maintenance, durability, and functionality.

Comfort vs. Performance

One of the most important balances in prosthetic use is between comfort and performance.

A highly dynamic prosthesis may offer:

- Greater speed
- More responsiveness
- Increased activity potential

But it may also require:

- More energy
- More precise control
- Greater physical conditioning

On the other hand, a more stable setup may:

- Feel safer
- Require less effort
- Be easier for daily use

But may limit higher-level activity.

The goal is not to choose the "best" prosthesis in general—it is to choose the best one for your current stage and goals.

These needs may change over time.

The Reality of Adjustment

Your first prosthesis will not be perfect.

In fact, adjustment is expected.

You may experience:

- Pressure points
- Skin irritation
- Changes in fit throughout the day

These are not signs of failure—they are part of the fitting process.

Your prosthetist relies on your feedback to make precise modifications.

Be specific when describing issues:

- Where is the discomfort?
- When does it occur?
- What does it feel like?

Clear communication leads to better outcomes.

Maintenance and Daily Care

A prosthesis requires regular care.

Daily habits should include:

- Inspecting your residual limb for skin issues
- Cleaning your socket and liners
- Checking for unusual wear or damage

Neglecting maintenance can lead to:

- Skin breakdown
- Poor fit
- Equipment failure

You don't need to overcomplicate it—but consistency matters.

Troubleshooting Common Issues

Over time, you may encounter challenges such as:

- Increased looseness or tightness
- Skin irritation or pressure sores
- Unusual noises or mechanical issues

When something feels off, address it early.

Do not wait for discomfort to become pain.

Small adjustments can often resolve issues quickly—but only if they are addressed promptly.

Your Prosthesis Will Evolve with You

Your needs today are not your needs forever.

As you progress, you may:

- Increase your activity level
- Improve strength and balance
- Set new goals

Your prosthesis should evolve alongside you.

This may involve:

- Component upgrades
- Socket replacements
- Changes in alignment

This is normal.

Your prosthetic journey is not static—it is adaptive.

A Closing Perspective

At first, a prosthesis may feel foreign, mechanical, and difficult to trust.

That is part of the process.

Over time, with proper fit, consistent use, and guided training, it can become something else:

A tool you rely on.
A system you understand.
An extension of how you move through the world.

You don't need to master it immediately.

You just need to begin learning—and stay engaged in the process.

Chapter 9

Learning to Walk Again

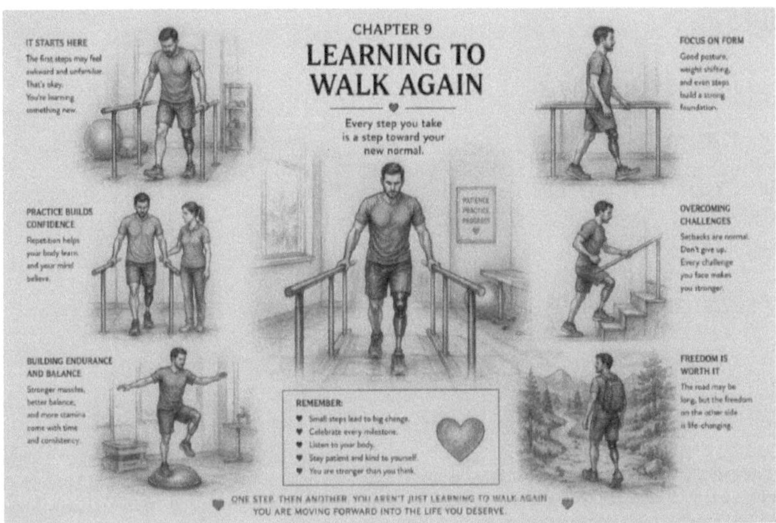

Learning to walk after limb loss is one of the most anticipated—and often most challenging—parts of recovery.

It is also one of the most misunderstood.

Walking with a prosthesis is not simply "picking up where you left off." It is a new skill. One that requires strength, coordination, patience, and repetition.

Progress will happen—but not all at once.

What Physical Therapy Really Looks Like

Before you take your first steps with a prosthesis, much of the work begins behind the scenes.

Physical therapy (PT) focuses on preparing your body for walking by building:

- Strength
- Balance
- Coordination
- Confidence

Early sessions may include:

- Standing balance exercises
- Weight shifting from side to side
- Core and hip strengthening
- Practicing proper posture

When you begin walking with a prosthesis, therapy becomes more structured.

You will work on:

- Gait training (how you walk)
- Step placement and timing
- Even weight distribution
- Controlled movement patterns

It may feel unnatural at first. That's expected.

You are not relearning your old walk—you are learning a new one.

The First Steps: What to Expect

Your first steps with a prosthesis can be a mix of emotions:

- Excitement
- Anxiety
- Uncertainty

Physically, you may notice:

- A feeling of heaviness or unfamiliar weight
- Difficulty trusting the prosthetic side
- Uneven or hesitant steps

You may rely heavily on:

- Parallel bars
- A walker or crutches
- Close supervision from your therapist

These supports are not setbacks—they are part of the process.

Your body and brain are learning how to work together in a new way. Stability comes before independence.

Building a Functional Gait

A "functional gait" means walking in a way that is:

- Safe
- Efficient
- Sustainable

Your therapist will help you focus on:

- Keeping your posture upright
- Taking even steps

- Avoiding compensations (like leaning or overusing one side)

Compensations may feel easier in the short term, but they can lead to:

- Pain
- Fatigue
- Long-term joint issues

Developing good habits early is critical—even if it feels slower.

Quality matters more than speed.

Milestones and Setbacks

Progress in walking does not happen in a straight line.

You may experience:

- Days where walking feels smoother and more natural
- Days where everything feels difficult again

Common milestones might include:

- Standing confidently with your prosthesis
- Taking independent steps
- Transitioning from walker to cane
- Walking short distances unassisted

Setbacks are part of the process.

They may be caused by:

- Fatigue
- Changes in limb volume
- Discomfort or fit issues

- Mental or emotional stress

A setback does not erase progress. It is a temporary fluctuation.

Assistive Devices: Tools, Not Limitations

Assistive devices are often used during the walking process.

These may include:

- Parallel bars
- Walkers
- Crutches
- Canes

Using these devices is not a sign of failure.

They provide:

- Stability
- Safety
- Confidence while learning

As your strength and balance improve, your reliance on these tools may decrease.

The goal is not to rush out of them—the goal is to use them effectively.

Energy and Endurance

Walking with a prosthesis requires more energy than natural walking.

You may notice:

- Faster fatigue

- Increased effort with longer distances
- The need for more frequent breaks

This is normal.

Energy demands vary depending on:

- Your level of amputation
- Your physical conditioning
- The type of prosthesis you use

Endurance builds gradually.

Short, consistent practice sessions are more effective than pushing too far and becoming exhausted.

Trusting the Prosthesis—and Yourself

One of the biggest challenges is trust.

You may hesitate to fully load your prosthetic side. You may unconsciously shift weight away from it or take uneven steps.

This hesitation is understandable.

Trust develops through:

- Repetition
- Safe practice environments
- Positive experiences

Each successful step reinforces confidence.

Over time, what once felt uncertain becomes more automatic.

The Mental Side of Walking

Walking is not just physical—it is cognitive.

You are thinking about:

- Where to place your foot
- How much weight to shift
- How to maintain balance

This level of focus can be exhausting.

As you practice, many of these actions become more automatic—but early on, mental fatigue is real.

Be patient with yourself.

Neural adaptation takes time.

Realistic Expectations

It's important to set expectations that are both optimistic and grounded.

You may not:

- Walk exactly the same as before
- Progress as quickly as you'd like
- Avoid frustration entirely

But you can:

- Improve steadily over time
- Build a safe and efficient walking pattern
- Regain independence in meaningful ways

Your path will be unique.

Avoid comparing your timeline to others.

A Closing Perspective

Learning to walk again is not a single moment—it is a process-built step by step.

There will be effort. There will be frustration. There will also be progress.

Every step you take—no matter how small—is part of something larger.

You are not just learning to walk.

You are rebuilding movement, confidence, and independence.

And that is worth the time it takes.

Chapter 10

Strength, Balance, and Mobility

CHAPTER 10
STRENGTH, BALANCE, AND MOBILITY
Building a strong body and steady balance helps you move with confidence and live life on your terms.
STRENGTH BUILDS CONFIDENCE
BALANCE IS EVERYTHING
FLEXIBILITY KEEPS YOU MOVING
MOVE YOUR BODY, CHANGE YOUR LIFE
MOBILITY MEANS FREEDOM
CONSISTENCY CREATES TRANSFORMATION
FOCUS AREAS
A STRONG BODY. STEADY BALANCE. GREATER MOBILITY
YOU HAVE THE POWER TO MOVE YOUR LIFE FORWARD.

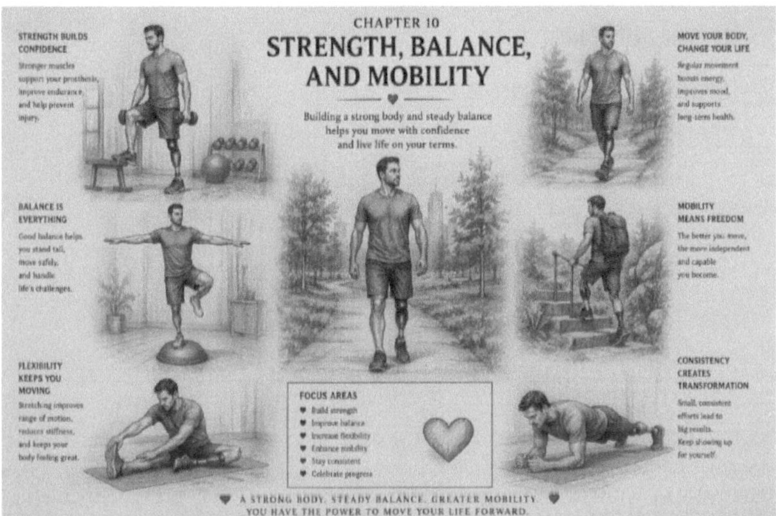

Walking is only one part of recovery.

Behind every step is a system of strength, balance, and control working together. Without that foundation, movement becomes inefficient, tiring, and potentially unsafe.

This chapter focuses on building the physical capacity that supports everything else—standing, walking, transferring, and eventually returning to higher levels of activity.

You are not just learning to move again.
You are building a body that can support that movement.

Foundational Exercises

Before advanced movement comes basic strength.

After limb loss, certain muscle groups often become weaker due to:

- Reduced activity
- Changes in movement patterns
- Time spent recovering

Key areas to focus on include:

- Hips and glutes (critical for stability and walking)
- Core muscles (for balance and posture)
- Remaining limb strength (for control and support)

Foundational exercises may include:

- Seated or lying leg raises
- Bridges for hip strength
- Gentle core activation exercises
- Upper body strengthening for transfers and mobility

These exercises may seem simple, but they are essential.

Skipping foundational strength often leads to compensations later.

Core Strength and Stability

Your core is the central stabilizing system of your body.

After amputation, the role of the core becomes even more important because your body must compensate for changes in weight distribution and balance.

A strong core helps:

- Maintain upright posture
- Control movement during walking
- Reduce strain on your back and joints

Core training does not require intense workouts.

It often involves:

- Controlled, intentional movements
- Maintaining alignment during exercises
- Building endurance over time

Even small improvements in core strength can lead to noticeable gains in stability and confidence.

Balance: Relearning Stability

Balance is one of the most affected—and most important—skills after limb loss.

Your body has lost a point of contact and sensory feedback. That means your brain must relearn how to:

- Distribute weight
- Respond to movement
- Maintain stability

Balance training may include:

- Standing with support, then gradually reducing it
- Weight shifting exercises
- Reaching tasks while standing
- Practicing controlled movements in different directions

At first, balance may feel unpredictable.

That is normal.

Balance improves through repetition and exposure—not avoidance.

Fall Prevention

Falls are a real risk during recovery—but they are also largely preventable with the right preparation.

Fall prevention involves:

- Strengthening key muscle groups
- Practicing safe movement patterns
- Learning how to recover from a loss of balance

Your therapist may work with you on:

- Safe ways to sit and stand
- Navigating uneven surfaces
- Turning and changing direction
- Strategies for getting up safely if a fall occurs

Confidence plays a role here as well.

Fear of falling can limit movement—but avoiding movement can slow progress.

The goal is not to eliminate all risk—it is to manage it effectively.

Building Endurance

Strength and balance allow you to move.

Endurance allows you to keep moving.

After amputation, you may find that even short periods of activity are tiring. This is expected.

Endurance is built gradually through:

- Consistent activity
- Increasing duration over time
- Allowing for recovery between efforts

This may include:

- Short walking sessions
- Repeated practice of daily tasks
- Light cardiovascular activity, as appropriate

The key is progression—not overexertion.

Pushing too hard too quickly can lead to:

- Fatigue
- Injury
- Setbacks

Steady, incremental increases are more effective.

The Role of Consistency

Improvement in strength, balance, and mobility does not come from occasional effort.

It comes from consistency.

You do not need perfect workouts or long sessions.

You need:

- Regular practice

- Intentional movement
- Follow-through over time

Even on days when motivation is low, small efforts matter.

Consistency builds momentum.

Listening to Your Body

As you increase activity, it becomes important to differentiate between:

- Productive effort
- Harmful strain

Some discomfort is expected when building strength.

But warning signs include:

- Sharp or worsening pain
- Persistent swelling
- Joint discomfort that does not improve with rest

Your body provides feedback.

Learning to interpret that feedback is part of long-term success.

Progress Beyond Therapy

Formal therapy sessions are important—but they are not the only place progress happens.

Real improvement occurs when you:

- Apply what you've learned outside of therapy
- Integrate movement into daily life
- Stay active in practical ways

This might include:

- Practicing standing while doing routine tasks
- Walking short distances at home
- Incorporating exercises into your daily schedule

Repetition in real-world environments builds functional strength.

A Closing Perspective

Strength, balance, and mobility are not separate goals—they are interconnected.

Each supports the others.

As these systems improve, you may notice:

- Greater confidence in movement
- Reduced fatigue
- Increased independence

Progress may feel gradual—but it is cumulative.

Every exercise, every repetition, every effort contributes to a stronger, more capable version of you.

You are not just recovering.

You are rebuilding.

Chapter 11

Protecting Your Sound Limb

CHAPTER 11
PROTECTING YOUR SOUND LIMB
Your sound limb does a lot of work.
Take care of it today,
so it can support you tomorrow.
THE IMPORTANCE
GOOD FOOTWEAR
STRENGTH AND FLEXIBILITY
MAINTAIN A HEALTHY WEIGHT
USE GOOD TECHNIQUE
STAY ACTIVE, STAY AWARE
DAILY CHECKS
LISTEN TO YOUR BODY
YOUR SOUND LIMB IS YOUR PARTNER IN EVERY STEP. CARE FOR IT, RESPECT IT, AND IT WILL CARRY YOU FORWARD.

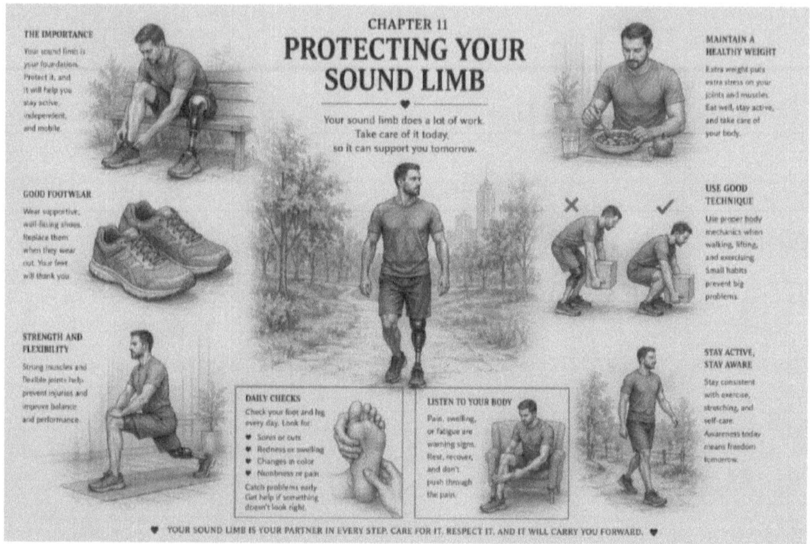

After limb loss, most of your movement, balance, and daily function shift to your remaining—or "sound"—limb.

It becomes your primary source of stability and power.

Because of this, it is placed under significantly more stress than it was before.

Protecting your sound limb is not optional.

It is essential for long-term mobility, independence, and quality of life.

Why It Matters More Than You Think

Your sound limb is now doing more work than it was designed to do alone.

This includes:

- Bearing more weight
- Compensating for balance changes
- Absorbing additional impact during walking

Over time, this increased demand can lead to:

- Joint strain
- Muscle fatigue
- Chronic pain
- Increased risk of injury

In some cases—especially for individuals with vascular conditions—overuse can contribute to serious complications.

Protecting your sound limb is not just about comfort today.

It is about preserving your mobility for the future.

Understanding Overuse

Overuse injuries develop gradually.

They are not usually caused by a single event, but by repeated stress without adequate recovery or support.

Common signs of overuse include:

- Persistent soreness
- Joint stiffness (especially in the knee, hip, or ankle)
- Swelling or inflammation

- Increasing discomfort during activity

Because your sound limb is used constantly, it can be easy to ignore early warning signs.

That is where problems begin.

Addressing small issues early prevents larger setbacks later.

Movement Patterns and Compensation

After amputation, your body naturally compensates.

You may:

- Shift more weight to your sound side
- Take uneven steps
- Rely more heavily on one side during transfers or standing

These compensations may feel helpful in the short term—but over time, they place uneven stress on your joints and muscles.

Physical therapy focuses on:

- Restoring balanced movement patterns
- Encouraging proper weight distribution
- Reducing unnecessary strain

Being mindful of how you move—even during simple tasks—can make a significant difference.

Footwear and Orthotics

Your sound limb depends heavily on proper support.

Footwear is not just about comfort—it is about protection and alignment.

Key considerations include:

- Proper fit (not too tight, not too loose)
- Adequate cushioning
- Good arch support
- Stability for walking and standing

In some cases, orthotics (custom or over-the-counter inserts) may be recommended to:

- Improve alignment
- Reduce pressure points
- Enhance shock absorption

Worn-out or poorly fitting shoes increase the risk of injury.

Replacing footwear regularly is a practical, preventative measure.

Strength and Conditioning

One of the best ways to protect your sound limb is to strengthen the muscles that support it.

This includes:

- Quadriceps (front of the thigh)
- Hamstrings (back of the thigh)
- Glutes (hip stabilizers)
- Calf muscles

Stronger muscles help:

- Absorb impact
- Stabilize joints
- Reduce strain during movement

Balance training is equally important.

Improved balance reduces the likelihood of sudden, awkward movements that can stress your sound limb.

Weight Management and Joint Health

Body weight plays a significant role in joint stress.

Every step places force through your joints—particularly the knee and hip of your sound limb.

Maintaining a healthy weight can:

- Reduce joint load
- Improve mobility
- Decrease the risk of long-term joint damage

This is not about perfection. It is about reducing unnecessary strain where possible.

Monitoring Skin and Circulation

For individuals with conditions like diabetes or vascular disease, monitoring the health of the sound limb is especially important.

Pay attention to:

- Cuts, blisters, or sores
- Changes in skin color or temperature
- Signs of poor circulation

Early detection of issues allows for early intervention.

Daily inspection—especially of the foot—is a simple but critical habit.

Rest and Recovery

Protection is not just about activity—it is also about recovery.

Your sound limb needs time to rest and recover from increased demands.

This may include:

- Taking breaks during prolonged activity
- Elevating the limb when appropriate
- Alternating tasks to avoid continuous strain

Ignoring fatigue increases the risk of injury.

Rest is not a setback—it is part of maintaining long-term function.

Working With Your Care Team

Your rehabilitation team plays a key role in protecting your sound limb.

They can help you:

- Identify risky movement patterns
- Develop strengthening programs
- Recommend appropriate footwear or orthotics
- Address early signs of overuse

Regular check-ins allow small issues to be corrected before they become larger problems.

A Long-Term Perspective

Your sound limb is now one of your most valuable physical assets.

Protecting it is not about limiting your life—it is about sustaining it.

With proper care, awareness, and consistent habits, you can:

- Maintain mobility
- Reduce pain
- Extend your independence over time

A Closing Perspective

It's easy to focus all your attention on the limb you've lost and the prosthesis you're learning to use.

But your sound limb deserves just as much attention—if not more.

It supports you every day.
It carries the extra load.
It makes movement possible.

Taking care of it is not optional.

It is one of the most important investments you can make in your long-term recovery and quality of life.

Chapter 12

You Are Not Alone

WE UNDERSTAND
CHAPTER 12
YOU ARE NOT ALONE
There is strength in connection.
There is hope in community.
There is a place for you here.
SHARE. LISTEN. HEAL. GROW.
COMMUNITY GIVES YOU STRENGTH
YOU HAVE PEOPLE WHO CARE ABOUT YOU
RESOURCES ARE THERE FOR YOU
REMEMBER
It's okay to ask for help.
It's okay to have hard days.
It's okay to celebrate small wins.
You are stronger than you think.
You are part of something bigger.
You belong here.
YOUR STORY CAN INSPIRE OTHERS
YOU ARE NOT ALONE IN THIS JOURNEY.
TOGETHER, WE HEAL, WE GROW, AND WE THRIVE.

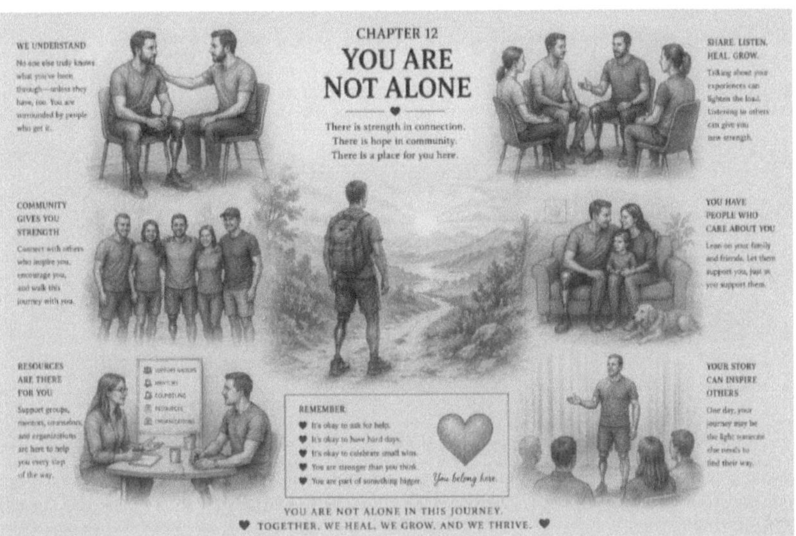

Limb loss can feel isolating.

Even when you are surrounded by supportive people, there may be moments where you think:

"No one really understands what this is like."

That feeling is common.

And it's also one of the most important challenges to address—because connection is not just helpful in recovery, it is foundational to it.

You are not the only person walking this path.

There is a community—whether you've found it yet or not.

The Reality of Isolation

After amputation, isolation can develop in subtle ways.

You may:

- Withdraw from social situations
- Avoid conversations about your experience
- Feel different from those around you

Even well-meaning friends and family may not fully understand what you're going through.

This gap in understanding can lead to:

- Frustration
- Loneliness
- A sense of being "separate" from others

Isolation is not just about being physically alone—it's about feeling disconnected.

And the longer it continues, the harder it can be to break.

Why Connection Matters

Human beings are not designed to recover in isolation.

Connection provides:

- Emotional support
- Practical guidance
- Perspective and reassurance

When you connect with others—especially those who have experienced limb loss—you gain access to something powerful:

Validation.

You begin to realize:

- Your thoughts and feelings are not unusual
- Your challenges are shared by others
- Your progress, even if slow, is meaningful

Connection reduces the sense that you are navigating this alone.

Finding Community

Community can take many forms.

You don't need a large network—you need the right connections.

Options may include:

Support Groups
In-person or virtual groups where individuals share experiences, challenges, and advice.

Peer Mentorship Programs
One-on-one connections with someone further along in their recovery.

Online Communities
Forums, social media groups, and virtual spaces dedicated to amputees.

Each offers different benefits.

Some people prefer structured environments. Others prefer informal, ongoing connections.

The format matters less than the presence of genuine understanding.

The Value of Shared Experience

There are certain things only another amputee can fully understand.

For example:

- The first time wearing a prosthesis
- Navigating phantom limb pain
- The emotional shifts that come with recovery

A peer who has lived this can:

- Normalize your experience
- Offer practical tips that professionals may not provide
- Share what helped—and what didn't

They don't replace your medical team.

They complement it.

And often, they provide reassurance in moments where clinical guidance alone is not enough.

Real Stories of Recovery

Recovery does not look the same for everyone.

Some people return to high levels of physical activity.
Others focus on regaining independence in daily life.
Many fall somewhere in between.

Hearing real stories helps you:

- Expand your understanding of what is possible
- Set realistic expectations
- See progress beyond your current moment

These stories are not meant to create pressure or comparison.

They are meant to provide perspective.

There is no single "right" outcome.

There is only your outcome.

Overcoming the Hesitation to Reach Out

Reaching out can feel difficult.

You may think:

- "I don't want to burden anyone."
- "I'm not ready to talk about this."
- "What if I don't relate to anyone?"

These concerns are valid—but they often keep people isolated longer than necessary.

You don't have to share everything right away.

You can:

- Listen before you speak
- Join a group without actively participating at first
- Connect with one person instead of many

Engagement can be gradual.

The important part is taking the first step.

Giving Back

At some point in your journey, you may find yourself in a different position.

You may:

- Have gained experience
- Developed coping strategies
- Reached milestones that once felt distant

When that happens, you may have the opportunity to support someone else.

Giving back can take many forms:

- Sharing your story
- Offering encouragement
- Becoming a peer mentor

Helping others does not require perfection.

It requires honesty.

And often, it reinforces your own growth.

Balancing Support with Independence

Connection is important—but so is maintaining your independence.

The goal is not to rely entirely on others.

It is to:

- Build a support system
- Use it when needed
- Continue developing your own capabilities

Healthy support empowers you—it does not limit you.

A Closing Perspective

If you feel alone right now, it does not mean you always will.

Connection may not happen immediately. It may take effort, time, and a willingness to step outside your comfort zone.

But it is available.

There are people who understand.
There are people who have been where you are.
There are people who are willing to walk alongside you.

You don't have to navigate this journey by yourself.

And you were never meant to.

Chapter 13

Returning to Life

CHAPTER 13
RETURNING TO LIFE
Life after amputation is not about getting back to who you were. It's about becoming who you are meant to be.
WORK & PURPOSE
You can build a career, pursue your passions, and make a difference.
DAILY LIFE
From the little things to the big moments, you've got this.
RELATIONSHIPS THAT MATTER
Surround yourself with people who lift you up, love you for who you are, and celebrate your wins.
STAY ACTIVE
Movement brings freedom, confidence, and joy. Find activities that challenge you and fuel you.
MAKE TIME FOR YOU
Do the things that bring you peace, joy, and fulfillment.
LOOK AHEAD WITH HOPE
The best days are still ahead. Keep dreaming, keep growing, and keep moving forward.
YOU'VE COME SO FAR
Be proud of your progress. Every step you take is a testament to your strength, courage, and determination.
You are resilient.
You are capable.
You are enough.
You are not defined by your loss.
You are defined by your courage to rise.
YOUR JOURNEY IS UNIQUE. YOUR FUTURE IS YOURS. LIVE IT FULLY.

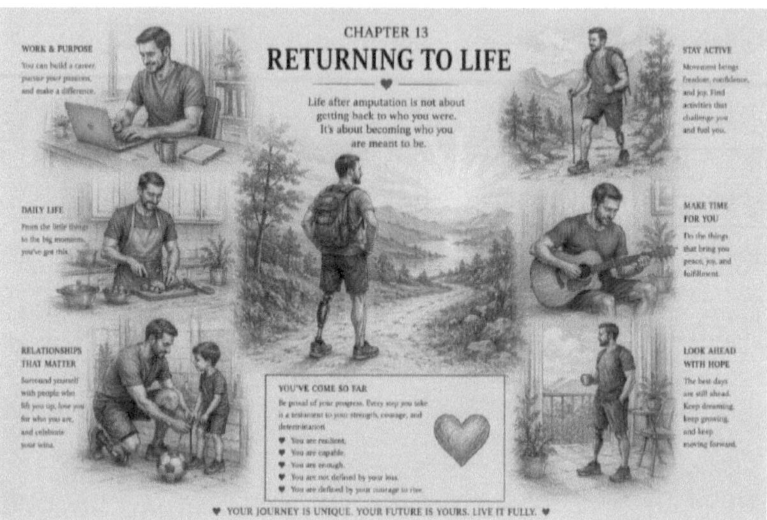

At some point in recovery, the focus begins to shift.

Early on, everything revolves around healing, therapy, and adaptation. But gradually, a new question emerges:

"How do I return to my life?"

Not the exact life you had before—but a life that is functional, meaningful, and fully yours.

Returning to life after limb loss is not a single event.
It is a series of transitions—practical, emotional, and social.

Work and Career Adjustments

Work is more than income. It often represents structure, identity, and purpose.

After amputation, returning to work may involve:

- Adjusting timelines
- Modifying responsibilities
- Learning new ways to perform tasks

Some people return to the same role with minimal changes. Others require accommodations or even a shift in career direction.

Common considerations include:

- Physical demands of the job
- Time required for recovery and rehabilitation
- Accessibility of the work environment
- Transportation and commuting

You may need to:

- Communicate with your employer about your needs
- Request reasonable accommodations
- Gradually transition back rather than returning all at once

This is not a step backward. It is a strategic approach to sustainability.

If returning to your previous role is not possible, this can be difficult—but it can also open the door to new opportunities that align better with your current abilities and long-term health.

Driving and Transportation

Regaining the ability to drive is a major milestone for many people.

It represents:

- Independence
- Flexibility
- Control over your daily life

Depending on your level of amputation, you may require:

- Vehicle modifications (such as hand controls)
- A period of retraining
- Medical clearance

An occupational therapist or driving specialist can help assess:

- Reaction time
- Coordination
- Safety

If driving is not immediately possible, alternative transportation options—such as rides from others, public transit, or ride services—can help maintain independence while you transition.

Relationships and Social Life

Relationships may feel different after limb loss.

You may experience:

- Concern about how others perceive you
- Changes in confidence
- Uncertainty about social situations

It's common to feel hesitant about re-entering social environments.

You might wonder:

- "Will people treat me differently?"
- "Do I need to explain what happened?"

The reality is: some people may not know what to say.

That does not mean they are judging you—it often means they are unsure how to respond.

You are not obligated to share your story with everyone.

You can choose:

- When to talk
- What to share
- How much detail to provide

Strong relationships tend to adapt.

People who care about you will adjust—not because you are different, but because the situation is new.

Intimacy and Personal Confidence

This is an area that is often overlooked—but it matters.

Changes in body image, confidence, and physical ability can affect how you see yourself in intimate or personal relationships.

You may feel:

- Self-conscious
- Uncertain about how to communicate your needs
- Concerned about acceptance

These feelings are valid.

Confidence in this area, like others, rebuilds over time.

Open communication—with yourself and with others—is key.

You are still capable of connection, attraction, and meaningful relationships.

Nothing about limb loss removes that.

Adaptive Sports and Hobbies

Returning to activities you enjoy—or discovering new ones—is an important part of reclaiming your life.

This may include:

- Adaptive sports (running, cycling, swimming, skiing)
- Recreational activities (hiking, fishing, fitness training)
- Creative or social hobbies

Adaptive equipment and techniques make many activities accessible.

Participating in these activities offers:

- Physical benefits
- Mental and emotional release
- A sense of normalcy and enjoyment

You do not need to return to everything immediately.

Start with what feels manageable—and build from there.

Redefining Independence

Independence may look different than it did before.

That does not make it less valuable.

Independence is not about doing everything exactly the same way.

It is about:

- Being able to meet your needs
- Making your own decisions
- Functioning in your daily life

You may use different tools. You may take different approaches.

But independence is still fully achievable.

Managing Expectations—Yours and Others

As you return to life, expectations can come from multiple directions:

- Your own expectations about progress
- Others' expectations about what you "should" be able to do

These expectations are not always aligned with reality.

Recovery timelines vary. Capabilities develop at different rates.

It is important to:

- Set realistic goals
- Communicate your limits
- Adjust expectations as needed

Progress is not about meeting external standards.
It is about building a sustainable, functional life.

Navigating Public Spaces

Being in public may feel different at first.

You may notice:

- People looking or asking questions
- Increased self-awareness
- Occasional awkward interactions

These experiences are common.

Over time, most people develop their own approach:

- Some choose to engage and educate
- Others prefer to keep interactions brief
- Some ignore attention altogether

There is no right way.

The key is finding what feels comfortable and sustainable for you.

A Closing Perspective

Returning to life is not about "going back."

It is about moving forward—with new tools, new awareness, and new capabilities.

There will be adjustments. There will be moments of uncertainty.

But there will also be:

- Progress
- Achievement
- Meaningful experiences

Your life is not on hold.

It is continuing—evolving in ways you may not have expected, but still fully capable of purpose, connection, and fulfillment.

You are not starting over.

You are continuing—differently, but still forward.

Chapter 14

Your New Normal

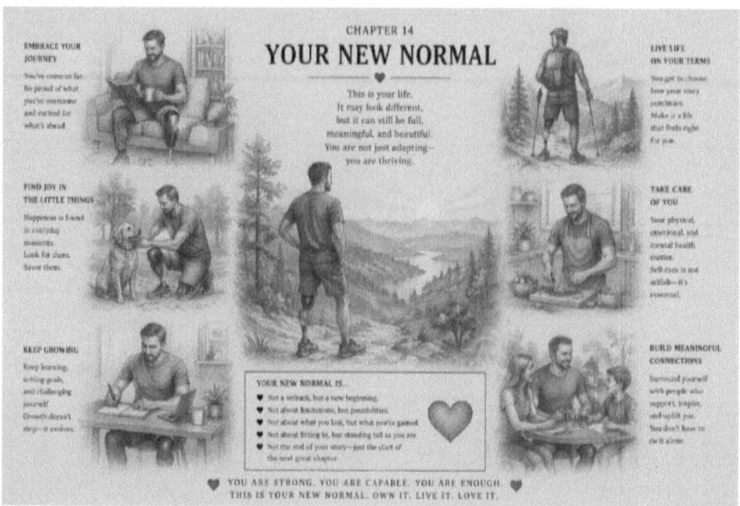

At some point in your journey, things begin to feel... different.

Not necessarily easier in every way—but more familiar. More manageable. Less overwhelming.

The routines you once had to think about become more automatic. The challenges that once felt constant begin to come and go.

This is where many people begin to recognize something important:

You are not just recovering anymore.

You are living again.

This is your new normal.

What "New Normal" Really Means

The phrase "new normal" can feel uncomfortable.

It may sound like settling—or accepting less than what you had before.

But that's not what it means.

Your new normal is not about lowering your expectations.

It's about redefining your baseline.

It reflects:

- What your life looks like now
- How you move, function, and engage with the world
- The systems and routines you've built

It is not static.

Your new normal will continue to evolve as you grow stronger, more confident, and more experienced.

Redefining Independence

Earlier in your journey, independence may have felt uncertain—or temporarily out of reach.

Now, it may begin to look more concrete.

Independence might include:

- Managing your daily routine
- Moving through your environment with confidence
- Making decisions about your care and lifestyle

It may not look exactly like it did before.

You may:

- Use assistive devices
- Take more time for certain tasks
- Approach activities differently

But independence is not defined by how you do something.

It is defined by your ability to do it in a way that works for you.

Confidence and Identity

Confidence does not return all at once.

It builds gradually—through repetition, experience, and small successes.

At this stage, you may notice:

- Less hesitation in movement
- Greater comfort in public spaces
- Reduced focus on limitations

Your identity also begins to stabilize.

Earlier questions like:
"Who am I now?"
may start to feel less urgent.

You are no longer trying to figure out who you are—you are actively living as that person.

Your identity now includes your experience—but it is not limited to it.

You are not defined solely by limb loss.

Living Fully Again

Living fully does not mean everything is perfect.

It means:

- You are engaged in your life
- You are participating in things that matter to you
- You are moving forward with intention

This might include:

- Returning to work or pursuing new goals
- Spending time with family and friends
- Engaging in hobbies or physical activities

There may still be challenges.

There may still be difficult days.

But they are no longer the center of everything.

Letting Go of "Before"

One of the most important—and often most difficult—parts of this stage is letting go of constant comparison to your past.

You may still think about:

- How things used to be
- What felt easier
- What you've lost

These thoughts may not disappear entirely.

But over time, they may carry less weight.

Letting go does not mean forgetting.

It means:

- Accepting that your life has changed
- Choosing not to measure your present solely against your past

Your life now is not a lesser version of what it was.

It is a different version.

Handling Ongoing Challenges

Even in your new normal, challenges will still arise.

You may experience:

- Changes in prosthetic fit
- Occasional pain or discomfort
- Periods of frustration or fatigue

These are not signs that something is wrong.

They are part of a long-term process.

The difference now is that you have:

- Experience
- Skills
- A better understanding of how to respond

Challenges may still occur—but they are more manageable.

Growth Beyond Recovery

At this stage, many people begin to experience growth that goes beyond physical recovery.

You may notice:

- Increased resilience
- A clearer sense of priorities
- Greater appreciation for progress and capability

Some people describe this as a shift in perspective.

What once felt overwhelming becomes something you know how to navigate.

This does not erase difficulty—but it changes your relationship to it.

Your Life Is Not Defined by Limits

It can be easy to focus on what has changed or what may be more difficult.

But your life is not defined by limitations.

It is defined by:

- What you choose to pursue
- How you adapt
- What you build moving forward

There are many paths to a meaningful life.

Yours may look different than you once imagined—but it is still yours to shape.

A Closing Perspective

Your new normal is not an endpoint.

It is a foundation.

A place where:

- You are more stable
- More capable
- More confident

From here, you continue forward.

You set new goals. You take on new challenges. You expand what is possible for you.

You are no longer just adjusting.

You are living.

And that—more than anything—is the goal.

Chapter 15

The Long-Term Journey

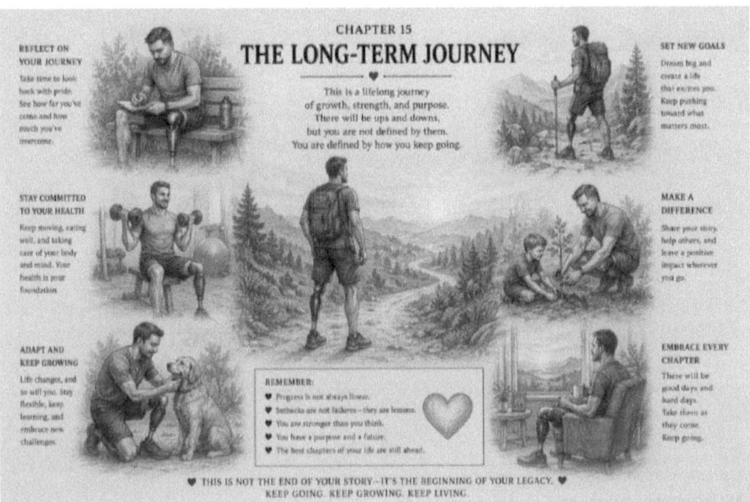

By this point, you've moved through the most intensive phases of recovery.

You've healed, adapted, learned new skills, and begun living your life again.

But it's important to understand something clearly:

Recovery from limb loss is not a finite process.
It is a long-term journey.

This chapter focuses on what comes next—not the early milestones, but the ongoing reality of living, adapting, and continuing to grow over time.

Prosthetic Changes Over Time

Your prosthesis is not permanent.

Even if it feels stable now, it will change—because your body changes.

Over time, you may experience:

- Fluctuations in residual limb volume
- Changes in muscle mass
- Wear and tear on components

This can lead to:

- The need for socket adjustments or replacements
- Upgrades in prosthetic technology
- Changes in alignment or fit

It's common for individuals to go through multiple prosthetic setups throughout their lives.

This is not a sign of failure.

It is a normal part of maintaining function and comfort.

Staying proactive—rather than waiting for major issues—helps ensure smoother transitions.

Aging as an Amputee

As you age, your body will naturally change—and those changes can interact with limb loss in specific ways.

You may notice:

- Decreased strength or endurance

- Changes in balance
- Increased joint sensitivity

These changes can affect:

- How long you wear your prosthesis
- How far or comfortably you walk
- Your overall activity level

The key is adaptation.

What works in one stage of life may need to be adjusted in another.

This might involve:

- Modifying activity levels
- Updating your prosthetic components
- Incorporating new support strategies

Aging is not a loss of ability—it is a shift in how ability is managed.

Protecting Long-Term Health

Long-term success depends on ongoing care—not just of your residual limb, but your entire body.

This includes:

- Maintaining strength and flexibility
- Protecting your sound limb
- Monitoring skin health
- Managing chronic conditions

Neglecting these areas can lead to:

- Increased pain
- Reduced mobility

- Secondary complications

Consistency matters more than intensity.

Small, regular efforts are more sustainable than short bursts of effort followed by inactivity.

Staying Motivated Over Time

Motivation often changes as you move further from the initial recovery phase.

Early on, progress is clear and frequent.

Later, progress may feel slower—or less noticeable.

This can lead to:

- Reduced consistency
- Frustration
- A sense of plateau

It's important to redefine motivation.

Instead of focusing only on visible progress, focus on:

- Maintaining function
- Preventing setbacks
- Continuing engagement in your life

Setting new goals can help:

- Trying a new activity
- Improving endurance
- Refining movement patterns

Motivation is not always about pushing forward aggressively.

Sometimes it is about maintaining what you've built.

Continuing Growth

Your journey does not stop at independence.

There is always room for growth.

This may include:

- Expanding your physical capabilities
- Exploring new hobbies or activities
- Taking on challenges you once thought were out of reach

Growth can also be internal.

You may develop:

- Greater resilience
- A stronger sense of identity
- A deeper understanding of your own capabilities

Limb loss changes your path—but it does not limit your potential for growth.

Adapting to Life Changes

Life will continue to evolve.

You may experience:

- Changes in career
- Family responsibilities
- Relocation or environmental changes

Each of these may require adjustments in how you:

- Use your prosthesis
- Manage your energy
- Approach daily tasks

Adaptability remains one of your most important skills.

The same mindset that carried you through early recovery will continue to serve you.

Revisiting Support Systems

Even in the long term, support remains important.

You may not need the same level of support as before—but maintaining connections can still be valuable.

This might include:

- Periodic check-ins with your care team
- Staying connected to peer communities
- Seeking guidance when new challenges arise

Support is not just for difficult times—it is also a resource for continued growth.

Redefining Success Over Time

Success will look different at different stages.

Early success might have been:

- Healing from surgery
- Standing or walking again

Now, success might be:

- Maintaining independence

- Staying active
- Living in alignment with your values

There is no single definition of success.

It evolves as you do.

A Closing Perspective

This is not the end of your journey.

It is the continuation of it.

You have already adapted to something significant. You have built strength, resilience, and capability.

Those qualities do not disappear.

They carry forward.

There will be new challenges. There will be adjustments.

But there will also be:

- Stability
- Growth
- Opportunity

You are not just someone who has gone through limb loss.

You are someone who continues to move forward—with experience, with awareness, and with the ability to adapt to whatever comes next.

Bonus Chapter

For Caregivers and Loved Ones

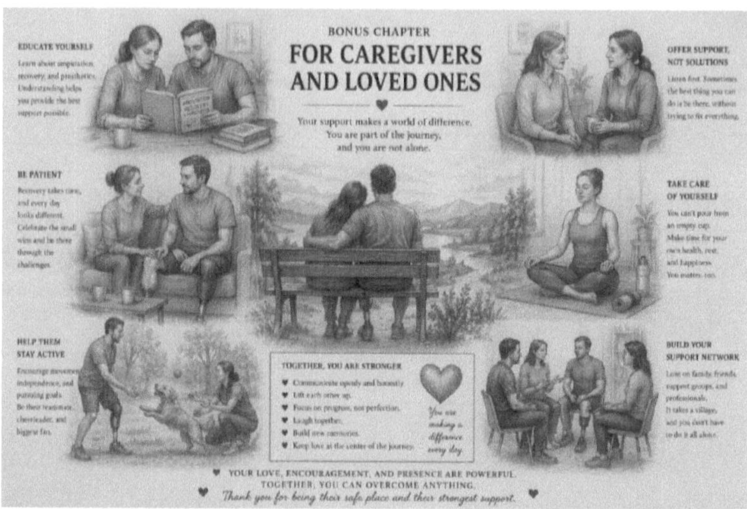

Supporting someone through limb loss is a meaningful and often demanding role.

You may feel a strong desire to help, protect, and ease their burden. At the same time, you may be navigating your own emotions—fear, uncertainty, frustration, or even grief.

This chapter is for you.

Because while the person experiencing limb loss is at the center of the journey, caregivers and loved ones are deeply affected as well.

And your role matters more than you may realize.

Understanding Your Role

You are not expected to "fix" everything.

You are not responsible for eliminating every difficulty or emotion.

Your role is to:

- Support
- Encourage
- Adapt alongside them

Sometimes that means helping physically.
Sometimes it means listening.
Sometimes it means stepping back.

The balance between support and independence is one of the most important aspects of your role.

How to Support Without Overstepping

It is natural to want to help as much as possible.

But too much assistance—especially when it's not needed—can unintentionally:

- Reduce confidence
- Limit independence
- Create frustration

A helpful approach is to ask rather than assume.

Instead of:
"Let me do that for you."

Try:
"Would you like help, or do you want to try it yourself?"

This gives them control.

Support should empower—not replace—their efforts.

Encouraging Independence

Independence is a critical part of recovery.

It builds:

- Confidence
- Skill
- A sense of control

Even when tasks take longer or look different, allowing space for independence is important.

This may require patience.

You may feel the urge to step in—but sometimes the most helpful thing you can do is allow the process to unfold.

Progress often happens through effort, not efficiency.

Communication: What Helps and What Doesn't

Clear, respectful communication is essential.

Helpful approaches include:

- Listening without immediately offering solutions
- Acknowledging their feelings without minimizing them
- Asking open-ended questions

For example:

- "How are you feeling about today?"
- "What's been the hardest part lately?"

Avoid:

- Dismissing emotions ("It could be worse")
- Forcing positivity ("Just stay positive")
- Comparing their situation to others

You don't need to have the right answers.

Often, being present and attentive is enough.

Understanding Emotional Realities

Limb loss affects more than the body.

Your loved one may experience:

- Grief
- Anger
- Frustration
- Moments of withdrawal

These emotions may come and go.

They are not personal attacks.
They are part of the adjustment process.

At times, you may feel unsure how to respond.

It's okay to say:
"I don't fully understand what you're going through, but I'm here with you."

That honesty builds trust.

Adjusting Expectations

Recovery is not linear.

There will be:

- Good days
- Difficult days
- Periods of progress
- Periods that feel stagnant

As a caregiver or loved one, it's important to:

- Avoid setting rigid expectations
- Recognize effort, not just outcomes
- Be flexible as needs change

Progress may not always be visible—but that doesn't mean it isn't happening.

Practical Support

There are many ways to provide practical help without overstepping.

This might include:

- Assisting with transportation or appointments
- Helping organize schedules or medications
- Supporting home modifications for accessibility

The goal is to reduce unnecessary stress—not to take over responsibilities completely.

Taking Care of Yourself

This is one of the most overlooked—and most important—parts of caregiving.

You cannot provide effective support if you are:

- Exhausted
- Overwhelmed
- Neglecting your own needs

Taking care of yourself is not selfish.

It is necessary.

This may include:

- Taking breaks
- Maintaining your own routines
- Talking to someone about your experience

You are also going through an adjustment.

Your well-being matters.

Recognizing When Additional Help Is Needed

There may be times when additional support is necessary—for both you and your loved one.

This could include:

- Mental health professionals
- Support groups
- Peer mentorship programs

Seeking help is not a failure.

It is a way to strengthen the support system.

Growing Through the Experience

While this journey is challenging, many caregivers and loved ones find that it also brings:

- Deeper connection
- Greater empathy
- A new perspective on resilience

You may discover strengths in yourself that you didn't know you had.

And your presence—your consistency, your willingness to stay engaged—can make a meaningful difference in your loved one's recovery.

A Closing Perspective

You don't need to do everything perfectly.

You don't need to have all the answers.

What matters most is that you:

- Show up
- Stay patient
- Remain willing to adapt

Your support does not need to be flawless to be effective.

It just needs to be real.

And in a journey like this, that is more than enough.

Bonus Chapter

Resources for New Lower Limb Amputees

BONUS CHAPTER
RESOURCES FOR NEW LOWER LIMB AMPUTEES
You don't have to navigate this journey alone. These resources, people, and tools are here to support you, empower you, and remind you that help is always within reach.
EDUCATION & INFORMATION
Learn as much as you can. Knowledge gives you confidence and helps you make informed decisions about your care and your future.
MEDICAL & REHAB CARE
FINANCIAL & LEGAL HELP
FINANCIAL ASSISTANCE OPTIONS
SUPPORT NETWORKS
ADAPTIVE TOOLS & TECHNOLOGY
EMOTIONAL & MENTAL WELLNESS
It's okay to not be okay.
SUPPORT
KNOWLEDGE
STRENGTH
HOPE
NEW BEGINNINGS
REMEMBER:
Ask for help.
Take it one step at a time.
Use the resources available to you.
You are stronger than you think.
Your new life is worth building.
YOU ARE NOT JUST RECOVERING—YOU ARE REBUILDING.
YOU ARE NOT JUST ADAPTING—YOU ARE THRIVING

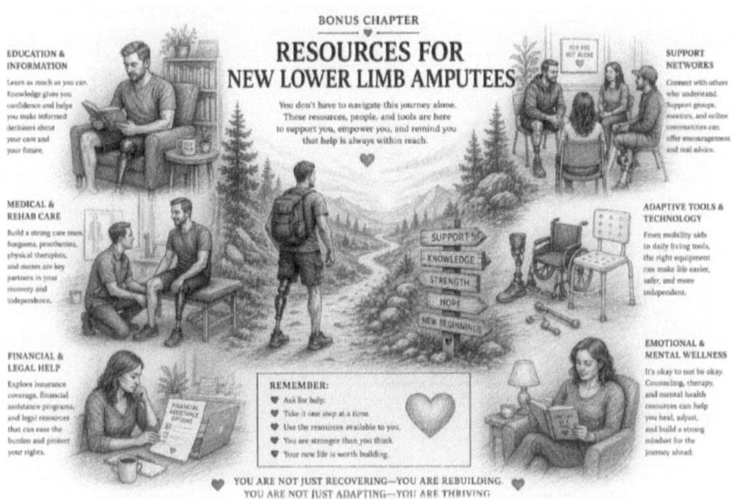

Navigating life after limb loss is easier when you know where to turn. The following resources provide education, support, financial help, and community connection to guide you through recovery and beyond.

1. National Organizations

Amputee Coalition

The most important starting point for new amputees in the U.S.

They provide:

- Education and recovery guides

- Peer support programs
- Support group directories
- Advocacy and insurance resources

National Limb Loss Resource Center

A centralized information hub connected to the Amputee Coalition.

Offers:

- One-on-onc information support
- (Phone: 888-267-5669; Email: wdoyle@amputee-coalition.org)
- Peer visitation programs
- Educational materials

2. Peer Support & Mentorship

AMPOWER

A nationwide peer mentoring network.

- Connects you with someone who has already gone through limb loss
- Provides real-world advice and emotional support
- Focuses on practical recovery and independence

Peer mentorship is one of the most effective tools for adjustment.

Support Groups (Local + Online)

Use:

- Amputee Coalition Support Group Finder

- Hospital-based rehab groups
- Online communities (including forums and social platforms)

Support groups help reduce isolation and normalize your experience.

3. Financial Assistance (Prosthetics & Care)

Limbs for Life Foundation

Provides financial assistance for prosthetic care.

- Helps cover costs for those without adequate insurance
- Offers guidance on navigating funding

Also serves as a referral source for additional amputee resources.

Additional Financial Help Sources

- Grants listed through the Amputee Coalition
- Nonprofits that recycle or refurbish prosthetics
- State disability programs

Financial support options exist—you often just need help finding them.

4. Rehabilitation & Medical Resources

U.S. Department of Veterans Affairs Amputation System of Care

Even if you are not a veteran, their materials are valuable.

Includes:

- Clinical guidelines for rehab
- Patient handbooks for lower limb amputation
- Long-term care frameworks

Rehabilitation Hospitals & Programs

Examples:

- **Shirley Ryan Ability Lab (IL)**
  Global leader in research-driven gait training and complex amputee care.
- **Kessler Institute (NJ)**
  Features advanced technologies like Computer-Aided Design (CAD) for socket fitting and robotic aids.
- **Spaulding Rehab (MA)**
  Offers specialized Prosthetic BOOST Therapy and adaptive sports for community reintegration.
- **TIRR Memorial Hermann (TX)**
  Renowned for upper-limb expertise and a formal partnership with the Amputee Coalition for peer support.
- **Brooks Rehabilitation (FL)**
  Provides extensive driver rehabilitation and adaptive equipment training to restore total independence.
- **VA Amputation System (National)**
  A massive network of 22 specialized sites providing veterans with advanced prosthetic and mental health services.

These centers provide:

- Physical therapy
- Prosthetic training

- Ongoing outpatient support

Rehab programs often include education, training, and support groups.

5. Education & Guides

Amputee Coalition “First Step” Guide

- One of the best beginner-friendly resources
- Covers recovery, prosthetics, and daily life
- Designed specifically for new amputees

Amplitude Magazine

- Articles, stories, and expert advice
- Resource directory with hundreds of organizations
- Covers lifestyle, prosthetics, and community

6. Community & Lifestyle Resources

Abilities Expo

- Events showcasing adaptive equipment
- Education and networking opportunities
- Exposure to new technologies and solutions

Adaptive Sports & Activity Programs

Challenged Athletes Foundation

- CAF grants support individuals with permanent physical disabilities that impair mobility, neuromuscular function, balance, or motor control.
- From beginners to Paralympic hopefuls, CAF grants are available for athletes of all ages and skill levels who meet eligibility requirements.
- CAF grants are need-based and available to athletes across the globe. Priority consideration is given to those without access to other funding sources.

Other Resources

- Local adaptive sports organizations
- Paralympic-style training programs
- Community recreation programs

These help rebuild confidence and expand what's possible.

7. Online Communities (Real-World Experience)

Online spaces can provide:

- Honest advice
- Shared experiences
- Daily encouragement

Examples include:

- Reddit amputee communities

- Facebook amputee support groups
- Organization-hosted forums

These communities complement—not replace—professional care.

8. Prosthetic & Clinical Resources

American Board for Certification in Orthotics and Prosthetics

- Helps you find certified prosthetists
- Ensures quality standards in care

Prosthetic Clinics (Examples)

- Martin Bionics
- Hanger Clinic
- Ottobock Patient Care
- ForMotion
- Local independent prosthetic providers

Your prosthetist is one of your most important long-term resources.

9. Global & Humanitarian Resources

LIMBS International

- Provides low-cost prosthetics and rehab
- Focuses on underserved populations

How to Use These Resources

Start simple:

1. Begin with the Amputee Coalition
2. Connect with one peer mentor or group
3. Identify your rehab team and prosthetist
4. Explore financial and lifestyle resources as needed

You do not need everything at once.

A Final Note

The most important thing to understand is this:

There is an entire ecosystem built to support you.

- People who understand
- Systems designed to help
- Resources you can access

You are not expected to figure this out alone.

You just need to take the first step—and know where to look next.

Epilogue

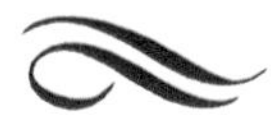

If you've made it to this point, take a moment.

Pause. Reflect. Breathe.

Because this journey—whether you're just beginning it or continuing forward—is not a small one. It takes strength to face the unknown. It takes courage to keep going when things feel difficult. And it takes resilience to rebuild, adapt, and move forward in a life that may look different than you once imagined.

But here you are.

And that matters.

By now, you've seen that limb loss is not just a medical event—it's a life transition. It changes how you move, how you think, how you see yourself, and how you engage with the world. But it does not take away your ability to live a meaningful, purposeful life.

Your story is not over.
In many ways, it is just beginning.

There will be challenges ahead. There may be setbacks, adjustments, and moments where things feel uncertain again. That is part of the process. But so are growth, progress, and moments of strength that remind you of just how capable you are.

You will find your rhythm.
You will discover what works for you.
And you will continue to build a life that is your own.

It may not look the way it once did—but that does not mean it cannot be full.

Full of purpose.
Full of connection.
Full of possibility.

As you move forward, remember this:

You are not defined by what you've lost.
You are defined by how you continue.

And if there is one thing I hope you take with you from this book, it is this—

You are stronger than you think.
You are capable of more than you realize.
And you still have so much life ahead of you.

Keep going.
Keep growing.

And continue living your best blessed life.

Afterword

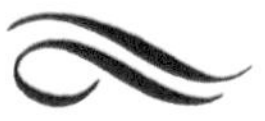

If you are reading this, it means you have taken the time to invest in understanding this journey—whether for yourself or for someone you care about.

That matters.

This book was created to provide guidance, clarity, and reassurance during a time that can feel overwhelming and uncertain. But no book, no matter how comprehensive, can replace your individual experience. Your journey will be your own—shaped by your body, your circumstances, your support system, and your mindset.

And that's okay.

Use what you've learned here as a foundation. Take what applies to you. Return to the sections that resonate most. Skip what doesn't. There is no single "right way" to move forward—only the way that works for you.

If there is one thing to carry with you beyond these pages, it is this:

You do not have to have everything figured out.

Progress happens over time.
Confidence builds with experience.
Strength develops through consistency.

Give yourself permission to learn as you go.

Also remember that support is not a sign of weakness—it is part of the process. Whether that support comes from your care team, your family, your peers, or your community, you are not meant to do this alone.

If this book has helped you in any way, consider sharing it with someone else who may benefit. The more knowledge and understanding we share, the stronger this community becomes.

And if you are in a place where you can give back—whether through encouragement, mentorship, or simply sharing your story—know that your voice has value. What you have experienced may be exactly what someone else needs to hear.

This journey does not end here.

It continues with each step you take, each challenge you face, and each moment you choose to keep moving forward.

Thank you for allowing this book to be a part of your path.

Acknowledgements

This book would not exist without the support, guidance, and inspiration of so many people who have been part of my journey.

First and foremost, I want to thank my husband, Damion. You have stood beside me through everything—multiple amputations, paraplegia, osseointegration, countless procedures, and the many challenges in between. Your strength, patience, and unwavering belief in me have been a constant source of support. Through every high and low, you never wavered. I would not be where I am today without you.

To my chosen family, thank you for your love, encouragement, and support throughout this journey. You have lifted me up in moments when I needed it most and reminded me of my strength when I questioned it.

To my caregivers, both personal and professional—thank you for your compassion, your dedication, and your willingness to show up every day. The care you provide goes far beyond the physical; it restores hope, dignity, and confidence.

To the practitioners and clinicians I have had the privilege of working with and learning from—your expertise and commitment to improving the lives of amputees is truly inspiring. Thank you for trusting me, teaching me, and allowing me to be part of this field.

A special and heartfelt thank you to Sara Peterson-Snyder, PhD, CPO, FAAOP(D), whose guidance and support were instrumental in bringing this book to life. From the earliest idea to the final printed pages, your expertise, encouragement, and belief in this project made all the difference.

To my colleagues and the team at Martin Bionics, thank you for your innovation, your support, and your shared mission to change the way prosthetic care is delivered. It is an honor to be part of a team that is making such a meaningful impact.

To the amputee community—you are the heart of this book. Your stories, your resilience, and your courage continue to inspire me every day. It is because of you that this work matters.

To those who have shared their experiences, asked difficult questions, and allowed me to learn alongside them—thank you. Your openness has helped shape the message within these pages.

And finally, to everyone who has encouraged me along the way—whether through a kind word, a shared moment, or simply believing in me—thank you.

This book is a reflection of all of you.

With gratitude,
Vaughan DeBarr

About the Author

Vaughan DeBarr is a bilateral above-knee amputee and paraplegic whose life story is a powerful testament to resilience, faith, and unwavering determination.

Her journey began with vascular disease resulting from trauma sustained during a pit bulldog attack in childhood—an experience that would shape the path she would one day walk with strength and purpose. In May 2013, she underwent a left below-knee amputation. In July 2017, that progressed to a left above-knee amputation. In June 2019, she became a bilateral above-knee amputee following the amputation of her right leg. Later that same year, on Christmas Day 2019, Vaughan experienced a spinal stroke at the L4/L5 level, resulting in paraplegia.

Through every stage of loss, uncertainty, and rebuilding, Vaughan chose to rise—not just for herself, but for others walking a similar path.

Since 2017, she has dedicated her professional life to the Orthotics and Prosthetics (O&P) field, where her lived experience brings a unique depth of understanding and compassion. As the Clinical Network Manager at Martin Bionics, the manufacturer of the innovative Socket-less Socket ™, she supports a growing network of four clinic locations and over 420 clinical network partners nationwide—helping improve the lives of amputees across the country.

In 2025, Vaughan took another courageous step forward in her journey by successfully undergoing osseointegration surgery, receiving OPRA implants by Integrum. She continues to work through intensive physical therapy with the goal of walking again using a cane—demonstrating that progress and possibility do not have limits, even in the face of extraordinary challenges.

Beyond her professional role, Vaughan is a passionate advocate, mentor, and voice of encouragement within the limb loss community. She actively participates in both professional and patient-centered events, sharing her story to inspire hope, strength, and possibility.

Known for always wearing cat ears in public, Vaughan carries a symbolic reminder that she has "nine lives." To her, it represents the courage to keep trying, to take risks, and to move forward without fear—because there is always another chance to rise. (Despite the symbolism, she doesn't own any cats.)

Vaughan's life is guided by her personal motto, "Living My Best Blessed Life." It is more than words—it is the way she chooses to face each day: with gratitude for how far she has come, courage to keep moving forward, and a deep belief that even through life's greatest challenges, there is still purpose, joy, and a life worth living.

www.ingramcontent.com/pod-product-compliance
Ingram Content Group UK Ltd.
Pitfield, Milton Keynes, MK11 3LW, UK
UKHW041639190726
13854UKWH00006B/2593

9 798995 883036